W9-CAJ-739

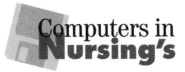
Computers in
Nursing's

Nurses' Guide
to the Internet

2ND EDITION

About the Author

Leslie H. Nicoll

Leslie H. Nicoll, PhD, MBA, RN is the Editor-in-Chief of *Computers in Nursing*, the only international peer-reviewed journal in nursing that focuses exclusively on computers, informatics, and technology, published by Lippincott-Raven Publishers, Philadelphia, Pennsylvania. In addition, Leslie is a Research Associate II at the Edmund S. Muskie School of Public Service at the University of Southern Maine. In this role, she serves as Principal Investigator and Project Director for HAPCEN: Hospice and Palliative Care Education Network, funded in 1995 by the National Cancer Institute, National Institutes of Health. She is an active member of Sigma Theta Tau, International Honor Society of Nursing, and the Eastern Nursing Research Society. She is a graduate of Russell Sage College (BS, Nursing), the University of Illinois (MS, Nursing), and Case Western Reserve University (PhD, Nursing). As a Commonwealth Fund Executive Nurse Fellow, she pursued MBA study at the Whittemore School of Business and Economics, University of New Hampshire, graduating in 1991.

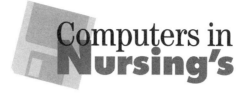

Computers in Nursing's

Nurses' Guide
to the Internet

2ND EDITION

Leslie H. Nicoll, PhD, MBA, RN
Editor-in-Chief, *Computers in Nursing*
E.S. Muskie School of Public Service
University of Southern Maine
Portland, Maine

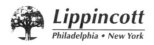

Lippincott
Philadelphia • New York

Acquisitions Editor: Lisa Marshall
Sponsoring Editor: Sandra Kasko
Project Editor: Barbara Ryalls
Senior Production Manager: Helen Ewan
Senior Production Coordinator: Nannette Winski
Design Coordinator: Nicholas Rook

Edition 2
Copyright © 1998 by Lippincott-Raven
Copyright © 1997 by Lippincott-Raven Publishers. All rights reserved. This book is protected by copyright. No part of it may be reproduced, stored in a retrieval system, or transmitted, in any form or by any means—electronic, mechanical, photocopy, recording, or otherwise—without the prior written permission of the publisher, except for brief quotations embodied in critical articles and reviews. Printed in the United States of America. For information write Lippincott-Raven Publishers, 227 East Washington Square, Philadelphia, PA 19106.

Materials appearing in this book prepared by individuals as part of their official duties as U.S. Government employees are not covered by the above-mentioned copyright.

9 8 7 6 5 4 3 2

Library of Congress Cataloging in Publications Data

Nicoll, Leslie H.
    Computers in nursing's nurses' guide to the Internet / by Leslie
H. Nicoll. — 2nd ed.
        p. cm.
    Includes bibliographical references and index.
    ISBN 0-7817-1435-4 (alk. paper)
    1. Nursing—Computer network resources.   2. Internet (Computer
network).   3. Nursing informatics.   I. Title.
    [DNLM: 1. Medical Informatics.   2. Nursing.   3. Computer
Communication Networks—nurses' instruction.   WY 26.5 N645c 1998]
    RT50.5.N53   1998
    025.06'61073—dc21
    DNLM/DLC   97-43982
    for Library of Congress   CIP

Care has been taken to confirm the accuracy of the information presented and to describe generally accepted practices. However, the authors, editors, and publisher are not responsible for errors or omissions or for any consequences from application of the information in this book and make no warranty, express or implied, with respect to the contents of the publication.

The authors, editors and publisher have exerted every effort to ensure that drug selection and dosage set forth in this text are in accordance with current recommendations and practice at the time of publication. However, in view of ongoing research, changes in government regulations, and the constant flow of information relating to drug therapy and drug reactions, the reader is urged to check the package insert for each drug for any change in indications and dosage and for added warnings and precautions. This is particularly important when the recommended agent is a new or infrequently employed drug.

Some drugs and medical devices presented in this publication have Food and Drug Administration (FDA) clearance for limited use in restricted research settings. It is the responsibility of the health care provider to ascertain the FDA status of each drug or device planned for use in their clinical practice.

Preface and Acknowledgments

Just 10 short years ago, or way back in 1987 (depending on your perspective), I was attending the Sigma Theta Tau Biennial Convention in San Francisco. In the Exhibit Hall was a staff member from the National Library of Medicine, demonstrating GratefulMed. GratefulMed is a software program that allows an individual to search the databases, such as MEDLINE, of the National Library of Medicine. On one hand, I was totally dismayed when I saw this program. I had defended my dissertation just 3 weeks before the conference. How I could have used this program while I was writing the proposal, conducting the research, and writing the final paper that became my dissertation! On the other hand, even though I had finished that component of my professional education, I knew that acquiring literature resources would continue to be part of my professional life.

I came home from that conference, ordered the software, and became connected to the online world. Although I had had a computer on my desk since 1983, this was the first time I was able to reach out, connect to another computer, and obtain information that was transmitted to me instantaneously. That first connection was the beginning of a profound change in how I carry out my day-to-day work.

The intervening years have brought many more changes. My first modem was a "zippy" 1200 baud; now I connect to the Internet through a high-speed cable modem connected to a cable television line (no more phone connection for me!). GratefulMed has gone from Version 2 to a Windows version (number 7) and an Internet version that is free to users throughout the world. Remember 10-megabyte hard drives? I am sitting here with a 2-gigabyte monster that is running out of room!

But the biggest change of all is the world of the Internet and the World Wide Web. Pictures have replaced text; videos, music, and more have brought my computer to life. Information pours through cyberspace and into my machine at a rate at which it is almost impossible to keep pace. It is clear that the explosive growth of the Internet is the most exciting new communication opportunity seen in my lifetime. At least, so far. Who knows where technology will take us next? When I think of the changes that occurred in just 10 years, it boggles my mind to imagine what technology will offer me in 2007.

Through this past decade of online exploration and investigation, I have become very comfortable with the Internet and the resources it has to offer. When I need information, I turn to the Internet first. This is true in my personal, as well as my professional life. I am sure that I am the first person in Maine to have Pergo® flooring, which I researched on the Internet and ordered from California. I had seen an advertisement in a magazine for the product but I could not find a store in the great state of Maine that sold it.[1] When my son needs to do research for a school paper, he turns first to the Internet. Even my husband, reluctant at first, has become an accomplished Internet traveler.

As Editor-in-Chief of *Computers in Nursing*, nurses have contacted me regularly to ask questions about Internet resources, information, or just how to get connected. I have learned that there are many nurses who are taking their first tentative steps toward discovering the world of online information and resources. They are enthusiastic but not sure where to begin. I have received repeated requests for information on sources and sites that would be of particular interest to nurses. People also asked me for suggestions of a useful guide or book that they could use to get started. After doing some research, I realized that such a guide did not exist. Thus the idea for the *Nurses' Guide to the Internet* was born.

When I finished the first edition in the spring of 1996, I thought my work was finished, for a while, at least. I should have known better. With the rapidity of changes occuring on the Internet, why should I expect a printed guide to be current for any great length of time? Even so, I was very pleased with the high level of positive feedback I received from readers of the first edition. Simple, concise, easy-to-read, "you make it clear for a novice" were some of the comments I received. I was happy that I had been able to provide necessary information to those who read and used the book, but I also realized that an out-of-date guide would not be much use to anybody. I took my cues from my readers and went back to the drawing board to update, revise, and expand the guide to bring you this completely overhauled second edition of *Computers in Nursing Nurses' Guide to the Internet*.

Although the content has been revised from top to bottom, some things have not changed. Just as with the first edition, the information included in this Inter-

---

[1]For those that are interested, you can learn more about Pergo at *http://carpeteria.com/ ~carpets/lam.htm* or *http://pergousa.com/.* It is also being sold in Maine now, at a number of stores.

net tour guide has been selected with an eye to efficient and rewarding professional Internet travel. The book is designed for nurses who have a desire and interest to "get on the Internet" but do not know where to start. In three parts I have provided three different types of resources: a general overview and user's guide that provides basic information (Part I); a comprehensive, cross-referenced index to the sites in the book (Part II); and an alphabetical directory of more than 510 sites, with addresses, contact information, and descriptions of each one (Part III). Every site has been visited, every listserv has been subscribed to—I have done my very best to bring you the most complete and current information possible. But recognizing that there will still be changes, a "late-breaking" information site has been established on the World Wide Web. Visit www.nursingcenter.com/books/isbn078-171435-4 to find out current addresses, changes, and new sites that have become available since this guide was printed. I hope that you find it useful in your work or maybe even *your* personal life.

This book is a natural outgrowth of the work I do as Editor-in-Chief of *Computers in Nursing*. It is a pleasure to have the strong support of my publisher at Lippincott-Raven, Lisa Marshall, and her very capable and talented staff. It is exciting to have a variety of methods with which to deliver the *Computers in Nursing* message to nurses around the world and the support of Lippincott-Raven Publishers to deliver that message. The print version of the journal, with its peer-reviewed articles, research reports, news, and reviews continues to break ground in the world of nursing informatics. *Computers in Nursing Interactive*, its online counterpart, has had a very successful start since its initiation in the summer of 1995. It continues to be a forum for late-breaking information, links to other sites, and a repository of content-rich resources related to nursing. This book, in combination with these resources, provides yet another vehicle to meet the computer information needs of nurses in all settings.

Earlier I mentioned my personal life. There are some very important people in my life who deserve my deepest thanks for their continuing and unending support—all of my family, but most especially my wonderful husband Tony and my loving and sweet children, Lance and Hannah. They are very proud of their mother and I am very proud of them! Even my pets—the ancient cats, Pookah and Bandit, and the newest member of our family, a retired racing greyhound named Jessie (check out the "Dogs" section of the Index)—help to bring a balance to my busy and sometimes overly hectic life. Thanks to all of you— and thank you, too, dear reader, for your support of my professional work.

Leslie H. Nicoll, PhD, MBA, RN

Contents

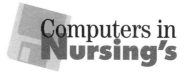

Computers in Nursing's

Nurses' Guide
to the Internet

2ND EDITION

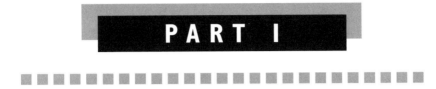

PART I

INTRODUCTION AND OVERVIEW OF INTERNET TRAVEL

CHAPTER I

■■■■■■■■■■■■■■■■■■■■■■■■■■■■■■■■■■■

Surfing Is Great . . .
If You Are on Vacation

HELLO, TRAVELER. . .

Welcome to the world of Internet travel. I have written this book to assist you as you begin your Internet journey. I have designed it to be a travel guide. Why did I decide to use that analogy? Well, I am assuming that if you are looking at this book, you have an interest in exploring the Internet. If so, you are about to embark on an exciting trip. Whenever I take a trip, I find that if I read a travel guide beforehand, I have a more successful adventure. But I bring the book with me, so that I know where the good sights are and how to find the best restaurants. I have discovered that Internet travel is no different. Although it is possible to dive right in and begin exploring, if you want to find specific material or particular types of information, your trip will be more rewarding with a handy travel guide. Thus, this book.

Lots of people talk about "surfing the Web" (short for World Wide Web or WWW) or "surfing the 'net" (short for "Internet"). Surfing is great, if you are on vacation. In fact, I have been known to while away many hours, surfing through the world of cyberspace. But there are times when it is necessary to put fun aside and buckle down to get some work done. Often, that work will require acquiring information and resources from the Internet. In that case, you are on a "professional trip," not vacation. In writing this guide, I am assuming that you are on either a business trip or a professional journey. Therefore, the information I have opted to include has been selected with an eye to professional, not vacation, travel. There are lots of Internet guides for the vacationing Internet surfer. There are not as many that deal with business travel for the professional nurse. This guide has been written to fill that gap.

A FEW ASSUMPTIONS

I am presuming several things about you, my reader. First, you are a nurse or, perhaps, a student studying to become a nurse. Either way, this book has been written with nurses in mind. Although other health professionals are welcome to read and use this book, I have geared the information in this guide to the needs of the working professional nurse. I know that nurses work in a variety of settings, doing a wide range of activities, in many different specialty areas. Using my experience, expertise, and interests, I have sought to include information that will be useful for the world of nurses with their wide range of professional pursuits.

Second, you are busy. Every day I experience the feeling of too much work and too few hours in which to accomplish it all. I imagine you have the same frustration. As you start on your Internet journey, I am assuming that you do not have time to waste. In fact, many people cite their lack of time as a barrier to becoming acquainted with the Internet—they believe that the time spent learning will not be rewarded with acquisition of useful information. Thus, I have tried to be concise to help you get started in a timely and efficient manner. Similarly, I have selected sites and resources to be useful and of interest to you as a busy professional. I have tried, as much as possible, to separate "the wheat from the chaff."

Nothing is more frustrating than hearing about a great resource on the Internet and then finding out it has been dismantled or, worse yet, abandoned by its developer. I have endeavored to select sites that are "going concerns," that is, sites that will be around for a while. An emerging phenomenon of the Internet is the fact that just about anybody with access can create a Web page, Gopher site, or a bulletin board, and put it "out there" for anyone else to see, use, or access. While this explosion of information is exciting, it has also led to lots of sites that are quickly rendered obsolete and never updated. Although I cannot guarantee that every Internet site included in the Directory of Sites will, in fact, be active when you go to access it, I have tried to select sites that appear to have a reasonable chance of survival on the Internet. In this way, this guide will help you to not waste too much time by visiting sites that no longer exist.

Third, you are a professional. As a professional, you want and need accurate, up-to-date information for your nursing work, but you also realize that you have a responsibility to assess the information that you obtain from whatever source. I am assuming that you use your critical thinking skills to verify all information you gather for your professional practice. Information obtained from the Internet is no different. For this guide, in selecting sites, I have chosen those that appear to be accurate, documented, updated, and contain useful information. I have done this by verifying dates when sites were created or updated, investigating the credentials of the site developer, and reviewing the material contained at the site. However, information on the Internet changes with the speed of light (or typing fingers on the keyboard). Therefore, even though I have done a preliminary screening, you must exercise your professional responsibility and personally assess information that you obtain from the Internet. As you visit sites listed in this guide, you will have the benefit of my assessment. But information may very well have changed between the time I visited the site and the time you do. Keep that in mind and do your own checking. Similarly, once you become familiar with Internet travel, you will be visiting sites that are not listed in these pages. You will need to develop your own criteria for evaluation, so that you can be assured that the information is truly useful and accurate for your work.

Fourth, you realize the value of information from a variety of sources. I hope to introduce you to the Internet so that it can become yet another component of your nursing armamentarium. But do not ignore other existing resources, including professional journals, books, libraries, audiovisuals, and publications from professional societies and organizations. The Internet is not the "be all and end all" of information. It is a useful resource, and it can bring to your desktop information that previously might have taken you days or weeks to find. Using the Internet can often save you a trip to the library or the cost of an envelope and stamp. But do not be fooled into thinking that all information is available on the Internet. It is not. As you become a seasoned traveler, you'll have a greater appreciation for what can be found where. Then you'll be in the best position to use your information resources wisely.

Finally, I believe that, as a nurse, you are adventurous, tenacious, creative, and patient. I have found these characteristics are often the defining feature of a successful nurse. To be an effective Internet traveler, you need to apply these same elements to your Internet journey. This book is a starting point, but you will encounter many situations where you are not finding the information or resources that you are seeking. If something is not working, think to yourself, "What does it take to solve this problem?" Do you need to try a little harder (tenacity), try a little longer (patience), or approach the problem in a different way (creativity)? I have found that each Internet stumbling block requires its own unique brand of problem solving. Keep that in mind so that you can enjoy your journey and not become frustrated when the answer is not immediate.

USING THIS GUIDE

As you begin your journey, I plan to offer you some keys to success that can make your trip more rewarding and productive. To meet this goal, I have organized this book in the manner of a traditional travel guide with three parts. Part I (which you are currently reading) includes a general overview of Internet travel. In the following chapter, I have included some "basic travel tips": getting online; necessary equipment; information on Internet addresses and language; and glossaries of helpful terms, abbreviations, and emoticons. The "site-seeing" guide in Chapter 3 includes an overview of the sites available on the Internet, a few caveats about what to expect and what not to expect, tips for effective searching, and information on making the transition from Internet traveler to Internet explorer. The user's guide for the Index and Directory of Sites composes Chapter 4.

Parts II and III form the core of the book. Part II is a comprehensive index that references Part III, "Directory of Sites." Parts II and III contain essential information for your Internet journey. In a traditional travel guide, these sections would be the hotel and restaurant listings; in this book, they include information on World Wide Web (WWW) sites, Listservs, Gophers, Usenet news groups, and telnet sites for remote login. Part II is a detailed, cross-referenced index that will tell you where to look in Part III (Directory of Sites) for the information you are seeking. To use the Index and Directory of Sites effectively, be sure to review Chapter 4. The Directory of Sites is arranged in strict alphabetical order, not by topic or specialty area. Listing the sites alphabetically facilitates finding a particular entry when you know it is there, but the alphabetical format makes it more difficult to find related areas of information. Of course, you can just browse through the directory and read the entries at your leisure. But if you want to find specific information, say, all the sites related to "cancer," then be sure to use the Index. The Index will point you to *all* the entries in the Directory of Sites related to a particular topic area. So don't ignore the Index; in some ways, it is the most important part of the book.

Enough introduction—let's get started on our trip!

CHAPTER 2

■■■■■■■■■■■■■■■■■■■■■■■■■■■■■■■■■■■■■■■

Basic Travel Tips

THE FIRST STEP: GETTING ONLINE

In the real world, the first step in any trip is to figure out how to get there: plane, train, bus, or car. Internet travel is no different. Your first step in Internet travel is to get connected, electronically, to the Internet world.

If you are connecting to the Internet solely through work or school, then you might not need to consider issues of hardware, software, and Internet connection. Someone else will have made these decisions, and you will be using equipment that is set up and ready to go. But maybe you don't have access through work, or you do, but you also want to be able to connect from home. If that is the case, read on. There are some issues you need to consider and important decisions you need to make.

Determining the type of Internet connection that is right for you requires some thought. Everyone immediately thinks hardware (what type of computer) and software are the primary concerns. However, your first step should be a quick assessment of your personal needs. You will be paying for an Internet connection, one way or another. Therefore, don't buy and pay for services you will not use. Consider your personal or professional communication requirements. Here are some questions to consider:

- Do you want to transfer files between computer systems throughout the world?
- Do you need to browse other computer systems such as those maintained by university libraries?
- Are you interested in exploring the new multimedia technologies that have recently flooded the World Wide Web (WWW)?

- Are you interested in sending electronic mail (e-mail) to friends and colleagues?
- What is your practice area? Are you practicing in a specialty area that requires up-to-the-minute practice information?
- Are you a student or nurse author, writing papers and manuscripts and needing literature resources?
- Are you a researcher who needs access to data and sources available online?

You may very well come up with a list of your own questions that will require some thought. Take your time and envision how you will be using your Internet access, because the answers to these questions will help you determine the type and kind of services you need from an Internet provider.

Connecting to the Internet requires a number of components, with several options, depending on the depth of service you need. The most useful approach is to try to find a variety of components delivered in one package, not multiple options for each. Even if you think you want access just for e-mail, it will not be long before you discover that you want some information that is available on the WWW. Therefore, you'll be better prepared if, at the outset, you try to establish a connection that will give you the greatest flexibility in adding or deleting services as you need them. More detail on options that are available will be presented later. For now, let's start at the beginning: hardware and software for Internet connectivity.

HARDWARE

Computers

There is not a computer being sold today that does not have the necessary components for accessing the Internet. The Internet has become so popular that all new computer buyers have this as a requirement, not an option. Does that mean you need to go out and buy a new machine? Not necessarily. Even an older personal computer can connect to the Internet without too much trouble. But the type of Internet services you can access will depend, to some extent, on how much computing power you have. An older computer with a slow modem will work just fine for e-mail or file transfer, but to really travel on the WWW, a much higher-end computer is required.

The WWW is made up of multimedia resources. World Wide Web browsers, such as Microsoft's Internet Explorer (IE) or Netscape, are based on graphical user interfaces. In other words, you see pictures and graphics, hear music, and read text. Programs such as these require a fast enough microprocessor, a big enough hard drive, and sufficient amounts of random access memory to run properly on computers with either Windows or Macintosh operating systems.

If you are buying a computer, take the time to do your homework. Read magazine articles in computer magazines such as *PC World* or *Byte*, and consult with your friends, colleagues, and knowledgeable salespeople to determine the best system for your needs. Remember this computer-buying truism as you begin shopping: buy the computer with the most computing power (microprocessor, random access memory, storage, video, and so on) that you can afford. Although it is often true that the computer you buy today will be obsolete tomorrow, you can do your best to stay ahead of technology by buying at the higher end, whenever possible.

If you are a total computer novice, you might want to spend some time using another computer to find out what you like and what works well for you. For example, if you take a college course, you may be able to use the computers in the college lab. There may be a mix of computers, including Macintoshes and PCs with Windows95. Which do you prefer? If you are not a novice, use your prior computer experience as a guide to what you should buy.

Necessary Equipment for Getting Connected

No matter what kind of computer you have, desktop or laptop, Macintosh or PC, your next step is to obtain the necessary equipment to make a connection to the Internet. Just a few years ago, you had essentially two choices: through a local area network (LAN) or by dial-in access through a telephone modem. Newer options, including cable modems and TV Internet devices, have recently become available.

NETWORKS

Most institutions connect to the Internet using a local area network. In this setup, each individual computer has an Ethernet card inside the machine, which allows the computer to connect to a local server. Each computer has a unique Internet protocol (IP) address. The local server provides the connection to a larger area network, often known as a WAN (wide area network). It is through these connections that you are able, from your desk, to communicate with computers all over the world. The actual technical configuration varies from institution to institution, but the concept is the same for any group of networked computers. The network connection is made through high-speed, fiber optic connections; you are not connecting through a telephone line.

MODEMS

The most popular way to connect to the Internet from a home or office standalone computer is through a modem. A *modem* is used to transmit digital information from a computer through ordinary phone lines to a network provider or Internet access provider. All modems work basically the same way and are generally packaged with the communication software needed to make them work. An internal modem fits into a slot inside the computer, whereas an external modem sits outside the computer with its own power supply and connects to the serial port on a PC or to the modem port on a Macintosh. The type you select can be a personal choice or may be dictated by your computer's configuration. As with buying a computer, if you do not own a modem, it is wise to consult knowledgeable friends or salespeople. Recent articles by Nicoll and Johnson have useful information for modem shoppers.[1,2]

Although there are many aspects to selecting a modem, perhaps the most important in terms of Internet access is speed. Modem speed is measured in bits per second (bps). A bit is the smallest amount of information a computer will recognize. The more bits your modem can send and receive, the faster the information will travel over the phone lines. Currently, modems that transmit at 56,600 bps, 28,800 bps, and 14,400 bps are available for purchase. Obviously, the faster modem is going to work better with the graphical user interface of Internet browsers, but by the same token, the fastest modem costs twice as much as the slowest! Keep this in mind when you go modem shopping.

Most modems sold today are fax-modems; in addition to communicating with other computers, you can send and receive faxes from your computer. Most modems come packaged with communication software, such as Bitcom or Pro-Comm, as well as fax software, such as FaxWorks or WinFax. If you are in a situation where you need to buy a separate communication software package, be sure it will support vt100 terminal emulation and Kermit or Zmodem file transfers. This ensures that your software can "talk" to the mainframe computer with which you'll eventually be communicating.

CABLE MODEMS

A fairly recent innovation are cable modems; these currently have limited availability in the United States, but the market is growing on a daily basis. A cable modem hooks to the cable line used for television, as opposed to the phone line, which is used by a traditional modem. The cable modem is an external modem with its own power supply. With a cable modem setup, you will need an Ethernet card in the computer (the same type of card used for a network connection). Two connections are made to the modem: the cable line (from the outside) and the network connection from the Ethernet card in the computer.

To take advantage of a cable modem, you must be in a location that has cable television. If the cable line is not available to your home (or office), then obviously you will not be able to make a cable connection. Cable modems are being installed and managed by cable television companies, such as Time Warner. Some companies do not require that you have cable television in order to have a cable modem, but some do. Similarly, pricing varies widely. Be sure to ask these questions if you are considering cable modem service.

A cable modem offers several advantages. It is much faster than a traditional modem; in fact, the speed is similar to that offered by a network connection. You will not be tying up your phone line while you are connected to the Internet.

And most companies offer unlimited access—you are not charged by the minute or hour while you are connected. So you can log on and surf to your heart's content without worrying about long-distance phone charges or connect charges through an Internet provider. Prices, while more expensive than providers such as America Online, are generally competitive. The big disadvantage is that you must have cable access, and your cable company must offer this service.

SATELLITE INTERNET ACCESS

Even newer than cable modems is satellite Internet access, which uses the same type of technology as for satellite television reception. A satellite is placed on your roof (or in your yard), and a card is inserted into your computer. If you already have a satellite, it may be possible to upgrade it to make the Internet connection; not all existing satellites can be upgraded. The computer connects to the Internet through the satellite. The service is supposed to be very fast—faster than a traditional modem or even a cable modem—although early tests indicate that the service might not quite live up to its claims in this department. It is also very expensive—you need to buy a satellite, pay for installation, and then pay a monthly access charge. If you want to have satellite television, that is a separate charge from the Internet service. Right now, the service is so new and expensive that it is probably not a realistic option for many people. However, as it becomes more popular and widely available, the price will probably drop. For people who live in locales where cable television and thus cable lines are unavailable, satellite connections may become a realistic option for fast Internet access.

INTERNET TELEVISION

The final option currently available is Internet television. This is actually quite different from the preceding discussion, because you are not buying a computer. Instead, you buy a device that sits on top of your television and brings the Internet to your home through your TV and phone line. These devices range in price from $200 to $500—definitely much less than buying a new computer system. With such a connection, you are able to access the Internet and WWW, send and receive e-mail, and read the news groups. Since it is not a computer, you will not be able to do any other computer activities, such as word processing, desktop publishing, or game playing. The manufacturers of Internet television devices make it clear that these are not a replacement for a home computer. But if you have a computer that is too old for upgrading for Internet access, but not so old that you want to get rid of it, Internet television might be a viable alternative.

Making a Connection: Access

INTERNET PROVIDERS

Once you have the proper equipment to make an Internet connection, your next step is to identify a provider for your access. Depending on what type of equipment you have, you may not have to make a decision. If you are connecting to the Internet through a network, then your access issues are solved. Similarly, cable modems, Internet television, and satellite Internet connections all come with access provision built in. However, in all likelihood, you will be connecting through a modem; if that is the case, you need to determine who will be your provider and how you will access the Internet.

If you are connecting with a modem, you will be dialing in to your provider through a phone line. Therefore, the following issues need to be considered:

- Long-distance versus local call
- Cost of the service
- Availability of connections

Selecting the best service for your needs may be a trade-off between these options.

Long-distance versus local call is a very important consideration. If you must make a long-distance call each time you make a connection, then, obviously, the longer you are online, the more the call will cost. For many people, this becomes cost prohibitive. For example, if you are a student at a university or college, you may be able to get a university account for Internet access at no charge. But if the number you need to call to make the connection is long distance, it may cost you more in the long run to connect this way. Commercial services, such as America Online or AT&T WorldNet, may be able to provide you with a local number or a toll-free 800 number. So even though you need to pay a monthly fee for the service, it may be cheaper than long-distance charges. The luckiest person is the one who has free university access and a local number to call. For many of us, however, this is just not the case!

If you are in a situation where both commercial service and university access are long distance or too expensive, do some research to find out what else might be available in your area. Perhaps a *FreeNet* exists in your community. FreeNets are gaining in popularity. These are community-based bulletin board systems with e-mail, information services, and usually at least some Internet services. FreeNets are operated under a concept much like public television, in that they are privately and community supported. They offer dial-in access and are, as the name indicates, free. How much Internet access they provide depends on the FreeNet, although most are adding more every day. Check with your local library—they may offer an Internet service, similar to a FreeNet, even if it doesn't go by that name.

A second option is to find a local access provider in your area or one that uses a local or 800 number for dial-in. Look in the yellow pages under "Internet Service Providers." Service provider rates vary greatly depending on the time of access, speed of access desired, and several other factors. It pays to shop around.

The final point to consider is availability. When your modem makes its call, it will be connecting to another modem at the other end. The number of modems available will determine if you get a connection or a busy signal. One of the advantages that commercial services like to advertise is the high rate of connectivity offered to their customers. If you have a local service provider, a limited number of modems may mean that it is very difficult to get through, especially at peak usage times. Even a university may have problems; the modem pool at the University of Southern Maine recently doubled its modem pool (from 30 to 60), but with the surging popularity of the Internet, a busy signal is still heard on a disappointingly regular basis.

Balance all three options together to make a final decision. Type of call, cost of service, and availability all need to be considered to arrive at a cost-effective and appropriate solution. What works for you may not be the same option chosen by your neighbor or friend, even if your computing needs are similar.

SOFTWARE

Once you have selected a provider, you need to determine your software needs. Again, many providers, such as America Online or Time Warner's Roadrunner cable modem service, include the software as part of the package. If they don't, however, or if you want to select a different program, you will need the following software to take advantage of the graphical user interface:

- **World Wide Web browser**—a hypertext markup language (HTML) browser that allows users to access World Wide Web home pages. Internet Explorer and Netscape are the most widely known as of this writing.
- **TCP/IP Stack**—TCP/IP is the Internet's communication protocol. The TCP/IP stack is the software that, when loaded on a PC, interprets the information that is sent to and from the Internet.
- **SLIP/PPP or LAN drivers**—SLIP and PPP are two protocols that allow dial-up access to the Internet through a serial link over normal phone lines. The LAN driver is used to connect directly to your local area network.

In addition, if you want to send and receive mail, you will need an e-mail program. Internet Explorer and Netscape both come with mail programs built in, and AOL offers e-mail as part of its package, but there are stand-alone mail programs available. Eudora, made by Qualcomm, is one such program. The "light" version is available at no charge and can be downloaded from the Internet.

Learning to Read the Street Signs

Just like in the real world, the virtual world requires addresses to navigate. To find your way around, you need an understanding of how Internet addresses work.

Today's Internet uses three addressing schemes:

- Domain Name System (DNS)
- E-mail
- Universal Resource Locator (URL)

Each type of address has a specific purpose. Let us begin with the DNS, which is the foundation of all Internet addresses.

Every computer node attached to the Internet has a unique numerical address known as an IP address. To the computer, it would look something like this: 129.237.28.3. Unfortunately, most of us have trouble remembering numerical sequences, particularly with more than 7 digits. This is where the DNS comes to the rescue. A name server translates an IP address into a text or name address like this:

MUSKIE2.USM.MAINE.EDU

This represents a node, which is a specific computer. Like your street address, each part has a specific meaning. From left to right the address goes from specific to general, just like your street address goes from top to bottom, specific to general. A DNS address breaks down like this:

MUSKIE2   The name of the local computer, in this case, it is a server for the Muskie School of Public Service at the University of Southern Maine.

USM   A subdomain, in this case, the abbreviation refers to University of Southern Maine.

MAINE   Another subdomain, here referring to the University of Maine.

EDU   The domain or type of institution.

The EDU extension refers to an educational institution. Others you may see include GOV for government, MIL for military, COM for commercial organizations, ORG for other organizations, and NET for network resources. Note that these extensions refer to addresses from the United States. For Internet travel outside the United States, there are a set of two letter domains, which correspond to the highest level domains for countries. For example, CA is Canada, UK is the United Kingdom, and ZA is South Africa. The United States has a country code (US) that is usually preceded by the state code (ie, ME.US for Maine). In the United States, most computers use the organizational domain names rather than the geographical name. Note that the two are not interchangeable. Using the example from above,

MUSKIE2.USM.MAINE.EDU

is not the same address as

MUSKIE2.USM.MAINE.ME.US

If you tried to send mail to the latter, it would be returned with a message, "unknown host address."

All Internet addresses, regardless of the interface used, are based on the DNS.

An e-mail address has two parts, a user identification (user ID) and a node, joined together by the @ sign. Sometimes the address can look as simple as

LNICOLL@MAINE.MAINE.EDU

where the user ID is LNICOLL and the node is MAINE.MAINE.EDU (which is one of the nodes for the University of Maine). Sometimes an address can be filled with odd symbols like !% or similar characters designed to guide the message between various smaller local area networks.

The URL is the "new kid" in cyberspace. Developed in Switzerland to navigate the WWW, the URL is rapidly becoming the standardized addressing scheme. Bear in mind that URLs require the use of a Web browser. A typical URL looks like this:

http://www.cini.com/cin/cin.htm

This happens to be the address of the WWW site for *Computers in Nursing Interactive*.

As with other Internet addresses, there is a method to what appears at first glance to be madness. It breaks down like this:

access_type://domain.name/directory_name/file.name

Using the *Computers in Nursing* URL mentioned above, the address is broken down as follows:

- http:// This represents World Wide Web access.
- www.cini.com In this case, the physical location is *Computers in Nursing Interactive*.
- /cin/ This is the directory path to a file called cin.htm, the home page for *Computers in Nursing Interactive*. Just what is a home page? I'll cover that in Chapter 3.

Other access types include:

- gopher:// To access Gopher sites.
- ftp:// To access FTP sites.
- telnet:// To initiate a telnet session.
- news: To access Usenet news. (Notice the absence of // for this access type.)

Learning the Language

The Internet world is full of *emoticons,* acronyms, and slang. The savvy traveler has an understanding of the language of the land. Although much of what is written on the Internet is in English, without some familiarity with the unique language of the Internet, you can quickly become confused as to what is really being said.

Display 2-1 is a glossary of common terms; Display 2-2 is a glossary of common abbreviations; and Figure 2-1 is a listing of emoticons. Abbreviations and emoticons, in particular, have taken on a life of their own on the Internet. Since

Text continues on page 20

DISPLAY 2-1.   GLOSSARY OF COMMON INTERNET TERMS

Application
1. Software that performs a particular useful function for you.   2. The useful function itself.

Archie
An electronic index of files found on anonymous file transfer protocol (FTP) sites. Keyword-searchable in both file name and description.

Backbone
High-capacity links that serve as the primary framework for the Internet globally.

Baud
When transmitting data, the number of times the medium's "state" changes per second. For example, a 2,400-baud modem changes the signal it sends on the phone line 2,400 times per second. Since each change in state can correspond to multiple bits of data, the actual bit rate of data transfer may exceed the baud rate.

Client
A software application that works on your behalf to extract some service from a server somewhere on the network. Think of your telephone as a client and the telephone company as the server to get the idea.

Dial-up
1. To connect to a computer by calling it up on the telephone.   2. A port that accepts dial-up connections.

Flame
A virulent and often largely personal attack against the author of a Usenet posting or e-mail message on a Listserv. Flames are unfortunately common. People who frequently write flames are known as flamers.

FreeNet
An organization to provide free Internet access to people in a certain area, usually through public libraries.

Gateway
A computer system that transfers data between normally incompatible applications or networks. It reformats the data so that they are acceptable for the new network (or application) before passing them on.

Gopher
A worldwide information service with many implementations, Gopher works as a top-level, subject-oriented menu system that accesses other information services across the Internet. It retrieves information from Internet connections and arranges it in a hierarchy, with each item representing either a file or a directory. The telnetting or FTPs are transparent to the user.

Internet
1. Generally, with a small "i," any collection of distinct networks working together as one.   2. Specifically, with a capital "I," the worldwide network of networks that are connected to each other, using the IP protocol and other similar protocols. The Internet provides file transfer, remote login, electronic mail, news, and other services.

Display 2-1. GLOSSARY OF COMMON INTERNET TERMS (CONTINUED)

Listserv

An automated mailing list distribution system enabling online discussions conducted by electronic mail throughout the Internet. The Listserv program was originally designed for the BITNET/EARN (European Academic and Research Network) networks.

Lynx

A text-only World Wide Web browser for any vt100 emulating terminal program using full screen, arrow keys, highlighting, and so forth. Fast navigation of cross-linked hypertext documents (not multimedia) over a low-speed dial-up connection. Originated at the University of Kansas.

NCSA Mosaic

Developed at the National Center for Supercomputing Applications (NCSA), Mosaic is a World Wide Web browser that allows easy point-and-click graphical hypermedia access to the World Wide Web over a SLIP (Serial Line Internet Protocol) or PPP (Point-to-Point Protocol) connection. Mosaic runs on Macintosh and Microsoft Windows and has integrated transparent access to all other Internet services.

Packet

A bundle of data. On the Internet, data are broken up into small chunks, called packets; each packet traverses the network independently. Packet sizes can vary from roughly 40 to 32,000 bytes, depending on the network hardware and media.

Port

1. A number that identifies a particular Internet application. 2. One of a computer's physical input/output channels (ie, a plug on the back).

Server

1. Software that allows a computer to offer a service to another computer. Other computers contact the server program by means of matching client software. 2. The computer on which the server software runs.

Service provider

An organization that provides connections to a part of the Internet.

Telnet

A protocol on the Internet that allows remote logins to another computer system. It is also a program that allows a user to browse menus, read text files, use Gopher services, and search online databases using the telnet protocol.

Usenet

A global bulletin board of sorts, in which millions of people exchange public information on a great variety of topics.

Veronica

A service on the Internet that maintains an index of Gopher items and provides keyword searches of those titles. The result of a search is a set of Gopher-type data items, which is returned to the user as a Gopher menu.

(continued)

DISPLAY 2-1.   GLOSSARY OF COMMON INTERNET TERMS (CONTINUED)

World Wide Web
The World Wide Web is a hypertext-based system that provides top-level access to various documents, lists, and services on the Internet. With a graphical user interface such as Mosaic, the WWW allows the creation and transfer of multimedia objects. It requires interactive access to the Internet.

Adapted from Hancock L. *Physician's Guide to the Internet.* Philadelphia, PA: Lippincott-Raven, 1996, with permission.

DISPLAY 2-2.   COMMON INTERNET ABBREVIATIONS

BITNET
Because It's Time Network. The grandfather of the Internet. BITNET is a mail-only network and is the primary source of discussion groups known as Listserv lists.

BBS
Bulletin board system.

BPS
Bits per second. The speed at which bits are transmitted over a communications medium.

BRB
Bathroom break.

BTW
By the way.

DNS
Domain Name System. An electronic mail addressing system used in networks such as the Internet and BITNET. The Internet DNS consists of a hierarchical sequence of names, from the most specific to the most general (left to right), separated by dots, for example, NIC.DDN.MIL.

FAQ
Frequently asked question.

FTP
File Transfer Protocol. The file transfer protocol is a method of sending files to and receiving files from a remote computer on the Internet. It is also the name of a program that uses the protocol to transfer files.

FYI
For your information.

<g>
Grin; often used in e-mail.

DISPLAY 2-2. COMMON INTERNET ABBREVIATIONS (CONTINUED)

GUI
Graphical user interface.

HTML
Hypertext Markup Language. Used to produce a hypertext document for display by a World Wide Web browser. HTML uses a standardized set of tags that tells the browser how to display the text as well as how to specify hypertext links.

HTTP
Hypertext Transfer Protocol. A protocol that defines hypertext links to information on the World Wide Web.

IMO; IMHO; IOHO
In my opinion; in my humble opinion; in our humble opinion.

IP
Internet Protocol. It allows a packet of information to traverse multiple networks on the way to its final destination.

LOL
Laughing out loud.

LAN
Local area network.

PPP/SLIP
Point-to-Point Protocol/Serial Line Internet Protocol.

RFC
Request for comments.

ROFL
Rolling on the floor, laughing.

RSI
Repetitive strain injury. Not technically a computer abbreviation, but it shows up quite a bit in discussion groups.

RTM
Read the manual. Often an "F" is inserted between the "T" and the "M." I will leave that abbreviation to the reader's imagination.

TCP/IP
Transmission Control Protocol/Internet Protocol. The basic protocol that allows information to be distributed over the Internet.

URL
Uniform Resource Locator. A standard for specifying the address of a document on the Internet, such as a home page, a file, or a newsgroup.

(continued)

Display 2-2. COMMON INTERNET ABBREVIATIONS (CONTINUED)

WAIS
Wide-Area Information Servers. A powerful system for looking up information in databases (or libraries) across the Internet.

WWW
World Wide Web.

Adapted from Hancock L. *Physician's Guide to the Internet.* Philadelphia, PA: Lippincott-Raven, 1996, with permission.

---

the majority of communications on the Internet are text based, that is, someone has to sit and type at a keyboard (even a graphic starts out as text), it only makes sense that abbreviations have become popular. Why type out "Frequently Asked Questions" when the acronym FAQ will do? For nurses, these abbreviations often have dual meanings. The abbreviation PRN (pro re nata), which means "as needed" to a nurse, means "printer" in the computer world. Other examples are OS/left eye/operating system, and CAD/coronary artery disease/computer aided design. Teeter and Wellman[3] have written an amusing article with more examples of nursing/computer terms; when you read it, it will be clear why you should not trust your nursing judgment to translate Internet acronyms!

Similarly, emoticons are very popular, especially in e-mail. Since e-mail strips away all the nuances of verbal communication, people often include little smiley faces to let someone know when they are to be taken lightly or are speaking "tongue in cheek" ;-). To see how an emoticon such as this works, turn your head sideways. Be forewarned: some people cannot stand emoticons; others sprinkle them liberally through all their messages. You'll soon develop your own style and will learn what is acceptable within your circle of e-mail colleagues.

The following list of emoticons comes from a site on the WWW at: http://wwws.enterprise.net/fortknox/emoticon/smiley.html#emot000

Full Version		Abbreviated Version
:-)	Happy	:)
(-:	Left handed/Australian	(:
:-(	Sad	:(
:-)	Winky/tongue-in-cheek	:)
#-)	Oh, what a night!	#)
:-O	Yelling/shocked	:O
:-I	Frowning	:I

For those wanting a more "aesthetically pleasing" emoticon you can use the profile version . . . some examples are below:

:^) :^(:^] ;^)

So, when words absolutely fail you . . . .

~:-[	Net flame	8-)	Wears glasses
:-$	Put your money where your mouth is	B:-)	Wears sunglasses on head
:-P	Sticking out tongue	:-T	Keeping a straight face/tight-lipped
:-@	Screaming/swearing/very angry/about to be sick	:-y	Said with a smile
:*)	Drunk/clown	:-I	Disgusted/grim/no expression
>;->	Wicked grin	:~-(	Crying/shed a tear
:-#	Been smacked In the mouth/wears a brace/kiss	:'-(	Crying
R-)	Broken glasses	:~(-~	Crying
(:-)	Bald	:-Q	A smoker
:-))	Is very fat	:-I	A smoker
:-{}	Wears lipstick	I-o	Bored
@:-)	Wears a turban	:-X	A kiss/lips are sealed
>:->	Leering	(:-D	Has a big mouth
$-)	Yuppie/just won a large sum of money	(:+)	Has a big nose
:'(	Crying	:-{	Has a moustache
:=)	Two noses	:-*	Just ate something sour/bitter taste/kiss
8:]	Gorilla	[:-)	Is wearing a walkman

FIGURE 2-1. Popular emoticons.

REFERENCES

1. Nicoll LH. Faxes, modems, and fax/modems. *Journal of Nursing Administration* 1995; 25(2):11–14, 22.
2. Johnson D. Modems: The gateway to cyberspace. *Computers in Nursing* 1996;14(4).
3. Teeter M, Wellman D. When is DOS not DOS? *Computers in Nursing* 1995;13(6): 301–302.

CHAPTER 3

▪▪▪▪▪▪▪▪▪▪▪▪▪▪▪▪▪▪▪▪▪▪▪▪▪▪▪▪▪▪▪▪▪

Site-Seeing Tips for the Internet Traveler

MODES OF TRAVEL DURING YOUR INTERNET JOURNEY

The Internet is a network of networks all working together to form a global community. The Internet uses unique addresses that can be used to locate information, and specialized software to let you virtually visit faraway places and move information around the world. Just as you need to decide whether to take a bus, drive a car, or ride a train on a traditional trip, you need to determine what mode of travel is appropriate on your Internet exploration. Different sites require different methods of transportation. This chapter is an introduction to different ways of travel and unique sites you can expect to see during your Internet journey.

Some people think that the Internet is a fairly recent development. Actually, the Internet has been around for almost 3 decades. It started out as a U.S. Defense Department network called the *ARPAnet* in 1969. Since then, it has grown, changed, matured, and mutated, but the essential structure of interconnected domains randomly distributed throughout the world has remained the same. As a matter of fact, ARPAnet no longer exists, but many of the standards established for that first network still govern the communication and structure of the modern Internet.

For many years, the Internet was more or less the private domain of scientists, researchers, and university professors who used the Internet to communicate and to exchange files and software. A number of events transpired in the 1980s and early 1990s that resulted in the enormous growth of the Internet and its ensuing popularity. Some of the changes were political, such as the High-Performance Computing Act of 1991, sponsored by then-Senator Al Gore; some were logistical, such as the decision to allow computers other than those used for research and military purposes to connect to the network; and some were just plain practical, such as the development of user-friendly software and tools that allowed less-experienced computer users to obtain information easily and quickly.

As I noted earlier, the first uses of the Internet were primarily communication and sharing of information. The tools used to accomplish these tasks were e-mail (for communication) and remote login, which had two functions: telnet (for browsing another computer) and file transfer protocol (FTP, for transferring files between computers). The original versions of the software for these tasks grew from either mainframe computer roots or Unix workstations. *Unix* is a popular operating system that was developed at the University of California at Berkeley. Unfortunately, both the mainframe systems and Unix require the user to learn a fairly arcane set of commands to complete even simple jobs. If you receive an e-mail message that is full of typos, weird spacing, and random letters, chances are the writer is struggling on a mainframe and having a tough time figuring out the editing commands needed to correct the mistakes. In recent years, a variety of software programs, such as Pegasus Mail or Eudora, Gopher, Mosaic, and Netscape, have all been developed. These programs are designed for the same original Internet activities of communication and information sharing, but they make the process much easier, allowing the more novice or casual computer user access to the same resources that the experts enjoyed for many years.

Internet travel is still based on e-mail and remote login, with its activities of telnet and FTP. When you use a program such as Netscape on the WWW, you may not realize that you are remotely connecting to another computer or using FTP to download files, but you are. It is possible to travel the Internet without knowing anything about how the system works, but you will find that if you have even a brief understanding of these tools, your trip is more likely to be successful. How you get around governs the sites and information that are available to you. Having an understanding of how you are getting around allows you to more efficiently find the type of information you are seeking. I realize that using traditional methods of remote login for telnet and FTP may be similar to riding a Concord coach across the country—slow, bumpy, and not very comfortable—but you'll eventually get where you are going. More pleasant travel is now possible, and you may never have to set foot in the "Concord coach" of remote login. But in case you do, a brief discussion of the grand ways of travel on the Internet follows.

Electronic Mail

By far, the most common use of the Internet is to send *electronic mail* (e-mail). It is also very easy. Exchanging e-mail with colleagues is probably the best way to become comfortable with the electronic world. Sending electronic mail across international networks is almost as easy as sending paper mail, but it arrives in seconds or minutes, rather than days.

To send e-mail you need two things: an address to send the mail to and a mail program. E-mail addresses are based on the domain name system discussed in Chapter 2. To obtain e-mail addresses, ask your friends and colleagues and begin an electronic address book. With the popularity of the Internet, many people include their addresses on their business cards. It is also possible to search for people on the Internet. A number of programs, such as Switchboard and Big Foot, have been developed for the express purpose of locating names, addresses, and e-mail addresses of people throughout the world. With a minimum of resourcefulness, you should be able to locate electronically connected long-lost friends and relatives, using the Internet.

You must also have a mail system of some sort. What is available to you depends on where and how you access the Internet. As discussed in Chapter 2, e-mail is one of the basic services provided by Internet access providers, so if you have Internet access, or are in the process of obtaining it, you probably have the tools necessary to send mail.

Different mail programs vary in their sophistication and complexity. Some include spell checkers; some do not. Cut and paste editing and retrieving files are common features in word processors but are not available in all mail programs. E-mail tends to be informal, and most recipients are tolerant of less-than-perfect communications. Words of warning: TYPING IN ALL CAPITALS IS NOT A GOOD IDEA. In popular *netiquette* (etiquette for the Internet) terms, typing exclusively in capital letters is considered shouting and very rude. Turn the caps lock off before you send your message.

Remote Login

Remote login means operating a computer, usually a mainframe, at a remote site from your home or office. It could be anywhere in the world. Originally, there were just two basic types of remote login: telnet and FTP. *Hypertext transfer protocol*, http, is the newest interface and is rapidly outpacing telnet and FTP. The popularity of http is making the need to type complex commands and know enough Unix to navigate the system a thing of the past. Even so, you may connect to a site where telnet and FTP are going on behind the scenes.

TELNET

Telnet is simply remote login and can be thought of as going to the library without a card—only browsing is available, and no files can be transferred. Telnet allows you to connect to a remote computer to search databases, read text, explore library catalogs, and much more. Login procedures are specific to each site. No uniform procedures have been established, but online help is usually available by typing "?" or the word "help." If you are using a browser, such as Netscape, when you initiate a telnet session, a second screen will pop up. It is from this screen that you navigate. Most telnet sites use some type of menu system to help the user navigate through the data. Telnet is all text based; you will not see any graphics.

An example of a popular telnet site is Fedworld (telnet://www.fedworld. gov), which is illustrated in Figure 3-1. Fedworld is an entry point into almost all federal government-maintained databases, including a dozen or so of interest to nurses, physicians, and other health care professionals.

Since telnet is like going to the library, it is not surprising that the majority of libraries that are connected to the Internet use telnet as their connection protocol. It is possible to log on and remotely search their card catalogs for their holdings. It may be possible to download the results of the search and e-mail the file to yourself, which you can then print and review off-line, at your leisure. Of course, to obtain a book from a remote library, you'll need to use interlibrary loan, if the title is not available to you locally.

Many libraries are changing over from being exclusively telnet based to having a hypertext (http) interface. If this is the case, you will be given a choice to choose the "graphical interface" or "text only version." The latter is usually the telnet connection. Why would someone choose a telnet connection? It may be faster and less cumbersome for searching, particularly if you are familiar with the commands.

When you search a library's catalog, you'll be searching a database that consists of the holdings of the library and includes materials such as books, theses, maps, and lists of journal holdings. Generally, the database will not include citations of journal articles. For that type of information, you need to search a specialized database, such as MEDLINE from the National Library of Medicine.

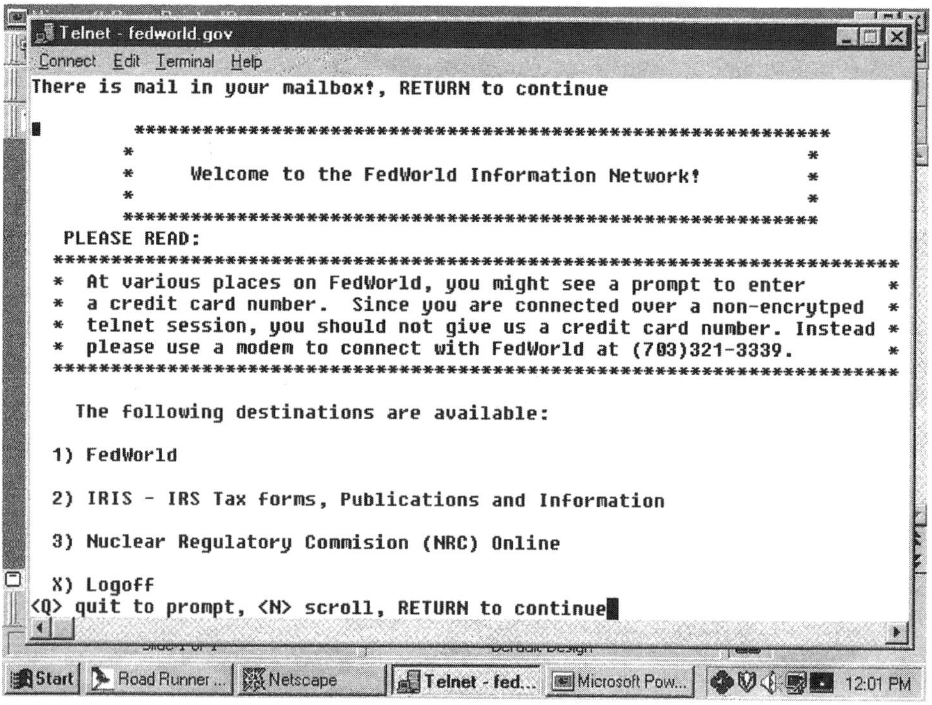

FIGURE 3-1. An example of a telnet site: FedWorld.

Many libraries offer access to the MEDLINE database, but if you log on to that library as an outsider, you may not be able to avail yourself of this resource. Why? Institutions that make MEDLINE and other similar databases available for their students, faculty, and staff pay royalty fees and contractually can allow only members of their institution to search for free. Thus, your access will be restricted via that route—but it is still possible to search MEDLINE and other databases remotely.

In the Directory of Sites, I have included entries for three databases that are available to you for searching for journal citations: Internet GratefulMed (IGM, to search MEDLINE); CINAHL Direct, and the UnCover Database of the Colorado Alliance of Research Libraries (CARL). A fee will be charged to use CINAHL; IGM and UnCover are free. There is a fee if you choose to order documents through UnCover, however.

CINAHL uses a telnet interface; IGM lets you search via the WWW using http; and UnCover gives you a choice. If you conduct sample searches in all three databases, you will have a good idea of the differences between telnet and http.

FILE TRANSFER PROTOCOL

File transfer protocol (FTP) is analogous to entering the library with a card. You are free to browse through a remote computer and take any public file of interest. File transfer protocol is used to transfer both text and binary (nontext) files over the Internet from one computer to another anywhere in the world.

There are two kinds of FTP sessions: personal and anonymous. To transfer a file to a colleague—a personal transfer—either the sender or the receiver must be authorized to log on to the other's account. Access to a personal account requires a password.

Anonymous FTP, which is open to the public, is so named because the login is the word "anonymous" (lower case and no quotes). The primary use of FTP is anonymous. Certain computer sites act as repositories of information and store vast numbers of files. There are more than 700 anonymous FTP sites open to anyone who has Internet access. These sites hold software for productivity and education, as well as informational text files, graphics, sound files, and movie clips.

File transfer, using FTP, works like this:

1. First, you log on to a local mainframe computer connected to the Internet.
2. Using FTP, a direct link is established to a remote mainframe computer, known as an anonymous FTP site.
3. You log in as anonymous; the requested password is usually your e-mail address. Most FTP sites are Unix based, so all commands, including anonymous, are case sensitive.
4. Once you are connected, you are able to look at directories and select files for transfer on the remote computer using the commands dir (directory) and cd (change directories).

5. When a file is selected, the command "get <filename>" will transfer the file to the local computer, for example, "get readme.txt."
6. Log off by typing "quit."

These basic commands will work on Unix-based FTP sites. Be aware that most, but not all, FTP sites use Unix. If you use FTP to a non-Unix site, the process remains the same but the screen will look different. Another complicating factor is that the FTP software or interface you use to connect to the site will affect the look of the screen and the steps needed to transfer the file. Some nice interfaces have been developed for the Macintosh (Fetch) and Windows (Ws-FTP) that provide a simple point-and-click file transfer. These programs require either a direct Internet connection or a SLIP/PPP type of connection.

HTTP

The final method of remote login is through *hypertext transfer protocol,* or http. This is rapidly becoming the most common way to navigate the World Wide Web. Telnet is text based; FTP is for transferring files. Hypertext transfer protocol takes advantage of graphics, movies, sound, and other multimedia resources. It allows you to click on a highlighted word or phrase (hypertext) and immediately be transferred to another location—perhaps even another computer. Again, this action is transparent to you, the user, but the language is how Internet navigation is largely handled.

In Chapter 2, I discussed the uniform resource locator (URL). Remember that the first part referred to access type, that is, **http://**www.cini.com/cin. When you see the URL in the address box on your browser, the access type will tell you what your computer is doing. Telnet and FTP are included as access types on the WWW.

SITES TO SEE DURING YOUR TRIP

Now that you have a basic familiarity with getting around, let us turn to sites that you will see. There is a world of sites out there; what you will see depends on what you are looking for.

World Wide Web

In the world of the Internet, some of the most exciting sites to see can be found on the World Wide Web (WWW). Commonly called Websites or the Web, this area of the Internet has grown exponentially during the past 5 years. The Web was created at the European Centre of Particle Physics (CERN) in Switzerland. These are the same folks who developed the uniform resource locator (URL). As you browse through some of the more peculiar sites on the Web, you may begin to wonder about the connection between the WWW and its physicist-creators in Switzerland.

As scientists engaged in research, they were constantly accessing and sharing files and data on the Internet and had been for years. But by 1989, the Internet had become unwieldy, even for them, the experienced users. The physicists were finding they were wasting valuable time navigating the Internet; this was cutting into the time available to them for their research. They decided to create an environment in which information of any type from any source could be accessed in a simple and consistent way. Their vision became the Web.

The key features distinguishing the Web from the rest of the Internet are hypertext and multimedia capabilities. Other Internet sites that I'll be discussing, including Gopher, Listservs, and Usenet groups, are all text based. The Web is full of color, pictures, sound, movies, and music. These are the features that have caught the public's attention and have in large part contributed to the phenomenal growth of the Web.

When you visit a Website, the first thing you'll see is the home page for that site. A *home page* is analogous to a welcome mat. Figure 3-2 is a picture of the *Computers in Nursing* home page. A home page will typically include information about the site, why it was created, what is available, and whom to contact with comments or questions. Home pages often include a running tally of the number of visitors *(hits)* and the date when the page was last updated.

The language used to create a Web page, *hypertext markup language* (HTML), has several advantages to developers and users. First, HTML can hold text formatting, which allows the designer to incorporate typical design elements into the page. This makes the page easy to read and attractive to look at. Second, HTML provides the ability to create hypertext links to other documents. As you move your cursor over highlighted areas within a WWW document, you'll see it turn into a hand or an arrow. By clicking on this area, using either a mouse or keystroke, another document will be retrieved and opened. This second document may be located in a completely different place on the Internet. Although the document could be on a computer in a remote part of the world, its physical location is irrelevant to you, the user. From the new document, you can click again to continue your exploration. Each of these clicks is called a *link.* As you travel the Internet using WWW links, you may end up in a different place, both conceptually and physically, from where you started.

With the proper helper applications, multimedia capabilities add a new dimension to Internet exploration. Graphics, sounds, and movie clips can be incorporated into a Website. While some of these sites are just plain fun (such as movie reviews[1]), there are also useful applications of multimedia. I recently met a faculty member who found a Quicktime animation of plaque building up on the arteries of the heart. She incorporated the video into a multimedia class presentation on coronary artery disease. Although the animation was only about 10

---

[1]There are movie review pages scattered all over the Internet, but one site that I particularly like is Mr. Showbiz at http://www.mrshowbiz.com.

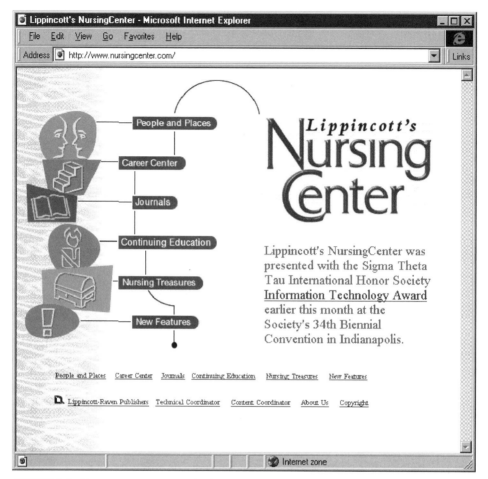

FIGURE 3-2. Visit www.cini.com on the Nursing Center Website.

seconds long, it clearly demonstrated for students a concept that is often hard to visualize.

The Web is also compatible with all other Internet tools (eg, Gopher servers, FTP, telnet, and Usenet). More important, because of the standardization developed for the HTML documents, anyone with access to a Web server can easily create a personal home page. For the first time in history, individuals can make information instantly accessible to any user worldwide.

To access the Web, you need a "browser" client. The original browser, Mosaic, was developed at the National Center for Supercomputing Applications (NCSA) in Illinois. It is available as freeware over the Internet and comes in Windows and Macintosh versions. One of the developers of Mosaic left NCSA, started Netscape Communications Corporation, and developed Netscape Navigator. This program, like Mosaic, comes in both Windows and Macintosh versions. Microsoft has also developed a browser, Internet Explorer. Netscape and Internet Explorer are fighting it out for user popularity; it remains to be seen which one will emerge as number one. Commercial services also provide access to the Web. If you have an account on America Online, for example, you can access the Web using its proprietary Web browser. The AT&T WorldNet service uses a modified version of Netscape; RoadRunner from Time Warner Cable uses a modified version of Internet Explorer. It is possible to have more than one browser on your computer, provided you have sufficient room on the hard drive. You are also not required to use a browser that comes with a program. For example, if you are an America Online customer, you can connect to AOL, minimize the browser supplied, and start your preferred browser, such as Netscape. Experiment with different programs to find out which one best meets your needs.

As noted in Chapter 2, to use any of these browsers satisfactorily, you must have an Internet connection through a LAN, modem, cable modem, or other connection and a relatively high-end computer.

Gopher

The WWW as we know it today was developed between 1989 and 1993 at CERN. Prior to that, the Microcomputer, Workstation and Networks Center at the University of Minnesota made the first serious attempt to bring a simple, practical user interface to the Internet with the development of Gopher software, which was introduced in 1991. The name is a bit of a joke: the software will "go for" (go-fer) your files. The University of Minnesota is also the home of the Golden Gophers. The software was made available free to educational institutions throughout the world. Because of their ease of use, Gopher servers rapidly spread throughout the Internet after the software was introduced.

Internet *Gophers* are information servers that present you with a hierarchical menu of resources in a simple, consistent manner. The advantage of using a Gopher server is that the software handles all the DNS addresses, as well as telnet and FTP commands. Internet navigation becomes a matter of reading menus.

Gopher is a client-server system. A Gopher "client" can reside on your personal computer or on a mainframe at your site, depending on how you access the Net. Gopher clients are also included in most Internet software packages. When the user selects menu options, the client connects to a remote Gopher server, which then presents the user with a series of menus for further exploration. Gopher also supports FTP for downloading files. Gopher's bookmark feature allows you to save site addresses in a file with the click of a mouse.

If you access a Gopher site through a browser, it is easily recognizable from the series of folders that are presented on your screen. An example of a Gopher site is presented in Figure 3-3.

University- and government-supported Gophers contain a wealth of medical- and health-related information, and publishers are starting to put their cata-

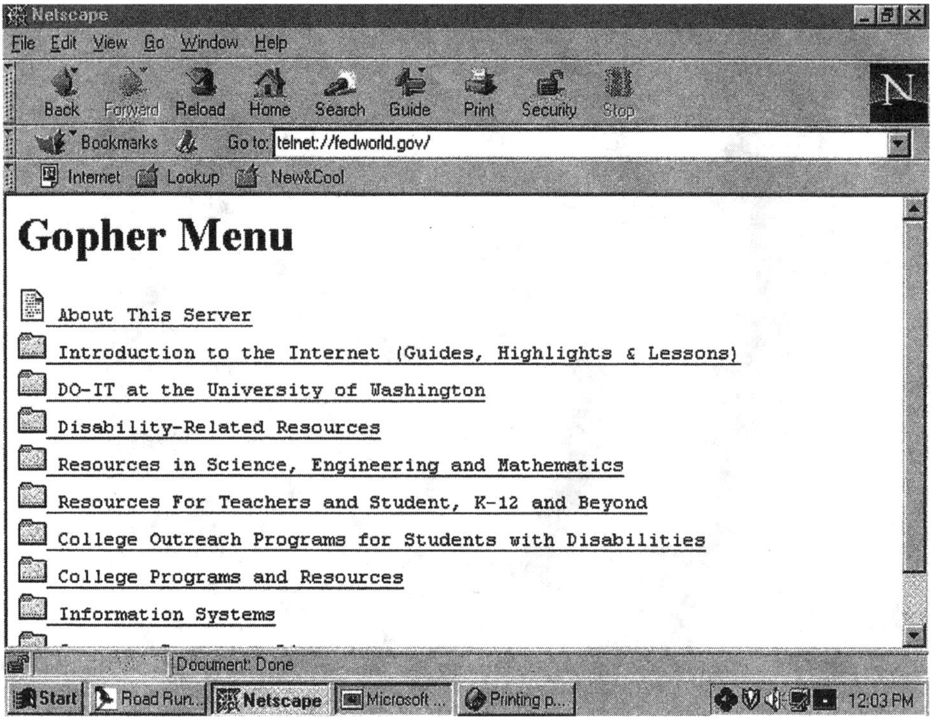

FIGURE 3-3. An example of a Gopher site: DO-IT Disability Resources.

logs on Gopher servers. One of the first nursing Gophers was the Nightingale Gopher at the University of Tennessee. This site was very well done with a wealth of information about conferences, people, and clinical issues. The site has been changed over to an http website, and the Gopher files are no longer available. Even so, we should remember the pioneering role that the Nightingale Gopher took when they first sought to organize and present nursing information to a wide audience of users.

Listserv Lists

SUBSCRIBING TO A LIST

One of the unique features of the Internet is discussion groups wherein the discussion is conducted by e-mail. The Internet has thousands of these special interest discussions, which are commonly referred to as *lists* or *Listservs*. There are several hundred health-oriented discussion lists concerning various specialties and diseases, and that number is growing rapidly. Using e-mail, you subscribe to a list electronically. Once subscribed, any mail posted to the list is distributed to all subscribers. Imagine asking 900 of your colleagues around the world a question concerning a clinical problem and receiving an answer within minutes, or discussing U.S. health care reform with health workers from other nations.

Generally, Listserv discussion groups can be divided into two types: layperson oriented and professionally oriented. An example of the former is the list AMPUTEE (to subscribe: Listserv@maelstrom.stjohns.edu), a forum to facilitate discussion among amputees, parents, children, relatives, and friends, as well as prosthetists, engineers, and other medical professionals. This list attracts people from all backgrounds, including many students. Professionally oriented lists include such forums as NURSENET (to subscribe: Listserv@listserv.utoronto.ca), a global forum for discussion of nursing issues, and NRSING-L (to subscribe: listserv@library.ummed.edu), a discussion group focused around nursing informatics.

To join a mailing list, you subscribe by sending the server an e-mail message. The format for subscribing is pretty standard from list to list. As an example, to subscribe to NURSERES, a discussion group concerning nursing research and related issues, you would send a message to LISTSERV@KENTVM.KENT.EDU. Leave the "from" and "subject" lines blank. Note that when you do this, your mail program may ask you if you intended to send the message with a blank subject line—answer yes. In the first line of the message, type: subscribe NURSERES <your name>; insert your name, such as Jane Doe, as you want it to appear on the subscription list. If you have an automatic signature added to your mail messages, turn that feature off before you send a subscription request. Figure 3-4 is an example of a completed subscription message. Once the message is received, one of the following will happen.

- You will automatically be added to the list, in which case you will receive a message confirming your registration and welcoming you to the group.
- You will be requested to send a confirmation; once the confirmation is received, you will be sent a welcome.
- Your name will be forwarded to the list owner for processing. Based on the decision of the list owner, you will (or will not) be added to the group.

High-volume lists usually ask for a confirmation message to be sent. Private or confidential lists often require screening. For example, AANURSES is a mailing list for nurses and other health care professionals in recovery. Because of the nature of the discussion and the goal of the list members to create a safe environment for its members, a person desiring to subscribe to the list must write to the list owner and describe the reason for wishing to join. Another wrinkle, just to keep you on your toes, is that this particular list has a slightly different method for subscribing. You send a message to AANURSES@ONTONSYSTEMS.COM. Put the word "subscribe" (no quotes) in the subject field. Leave the message blank. The list owner will contact you privately to confirm your subscription.

Once your subscription is successfully processed, you'll get an automatically generated message informing you that you are subscribed. You'll often get a message from the list owner, welcoming you to the group and telling you about

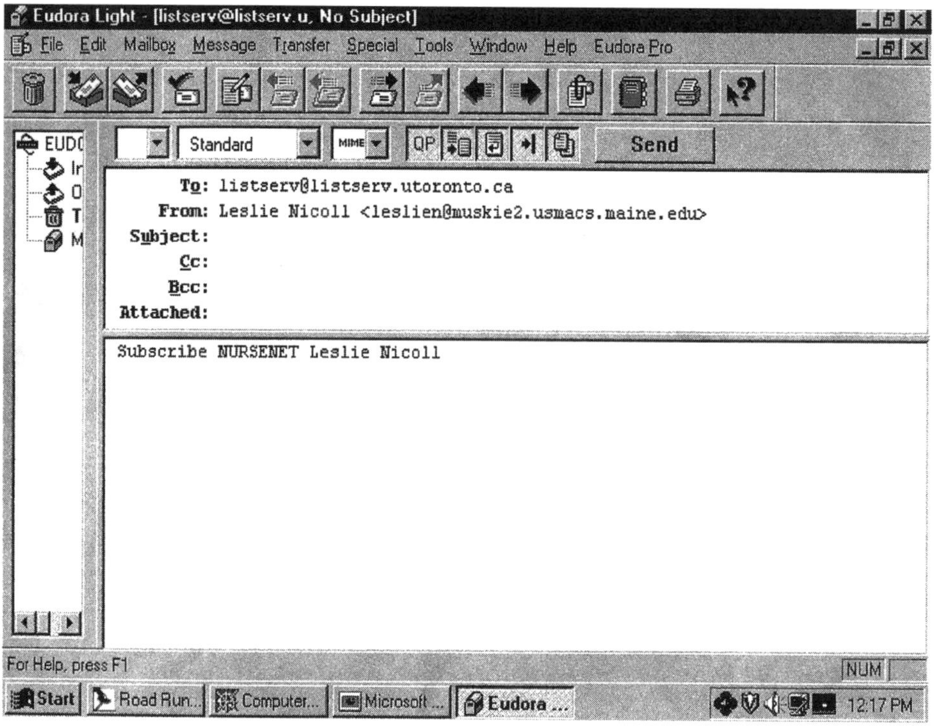

FIGURE 3-4. E-mail message to subscribe to a list.

list netiquette. The welcome message often includes helpful information on how to *unsubscribe,* or stop the mail, so you might want to print and save it for future reference.

Once you are a member of a mailing list, messages can be sent to all the subscribers by addressing the message to the group. For the nursing research group, the address is NURSERES@KENTVM.KENT.EDU. Be forewarned, some active lists may generate 20, 30, or more messages a day. If you are paying for a connection that charges for messages received, it could get expensive. If your mailbox is small, messages will bounce back to the list owner or the list, which is also a source of aggravation for the members.

All lists have owners, but that does not mean the list is moderated. In a *moderated discussion,* all messages go to the list owner before they are posted to the list. In an *unmoderated discussion,* the messages automatically go to the entire list. There are advantages and disadvantages to each. In a moderated list, all the error messages (the ones that say "How do I unsubscribe from this list?" over and over) will be deleted. Similarly, wildly inappropriate messages never make it to the group. On the other hand, some people find the moderating process to be uncomfortably akin to censorship. Which is better? You can decide after you experience both types of lists. Of the lists mentioned previously, NURSERES is moderated, NURSENET is not.

Closed lists also exist. A *closed list* is one in which the subscribers are restricted; for example, students registered in a particular class may be the only people able to subscribe to a list. Generally, the addresses of closed lists are not made public, but it is possible to search on a mainframe to find out the names of all lists that reside on that mainframe. If you try to subscribe to a list and your subscription is refused, it may be because it is a closed list.

How Do Listservs Work?

Listserv is simply a software application designed for e-mail distribution. The original Listserv software was written by Eric Thomas for the IBM mainframe VM/CMS operating system, although the term Listserv has evolved into a generic name for all e-mail distribution software that has been developed for various mainframe operating systems. It currently seems that only Internet purists distinguish between Listserv and the Unix Listproc and Majordomo software, or the UK's Mailbase program. Is this distinction important? There is, of course, the ethical consideration of crediting software titles and authors, but there is a second consideration for the user. Although all server software appears to be similar, there are important differences. For example, the "subscribe" command is the same for Listserv and Listproc, but to get a list of subscribers the command is "review" for Listserv and "recipient" for Listproc. You can usually figure out which software a system is using by the address of the list. For example, the NURSERES list is on a system using Listserv software (LISTSERV@KENTVM.KENT.EDU), NURSE-ROGERS is on a system using Mailbase (MAILBASE@MAILBASE.-AC.UK), NURSE-UK is a Majordomo system (MAJORDOMO@BHAM.AC.UK), PERIOP is on a Listproc system (LISTPROC@U.WASHINGTON.EDU), and PEDIATRIC-PAIN is on a Mailserv system (MAILSERV@AC.DAL.CA). Descriptions of all these lists are included in the Directory of Sites; a summary of the different mail server commands for the different programs can be found in Display 3-1.

A close cousin of Listserv groups are electronic publications. While they do not invite discussion, most are subscribed to and distributed in the same manner as the discussion groups. Many electronic publications are distributed free to subscribers across the Internet. They vary in frequency, but all offer timely information to the health and medical community, and most welcome reader interaction.

Usenet News Groups

Usenet news groups are topical discussion special interest groups, similar in many ways to Listserv discussion groups. Unlike Listserv lists, where one has to subscribe to receive messages by e-mail, the "posts" in the Usenet groups are stored

Text continues on page 39

DISPLAY 3-1. GLOSSARY OF MAIL SERVER COMMANDS

The following is a comparison of mail server commands for five different mailing list programs: listproc, Listserv, Mailbase, mailserv, and majordomo.

To join a list:

Listproc: **SUBSCRIBE [listname] Firstname Lastname**
(eg **SUBSCRIBE PERIOP** Jane Doe)

Listserv: **SUBSCRIBE [listname] Firstname Lastname**
(eg **SUBSCRIBE NURSERES** Jane Doe)

Mailbase: **JOIN [listname] Firstname Lastname**
(eg **JOIN NURSE-ROGERS** Jane Doe)

Mailserv: **SUBSCRIBE [listname] Firstname Lastname**
(eg **SUBSCRIBE PEDIATRIC PAIN** Jane Doe)
Optionally, include the e-mail address at which you wish to receive listmail.
(eg **SUBSCRIBE [listname] Firstname Lastname [address]**)

Majordomo: **SUBSCRIBE [listname]**
(eg **SUBSCRIBE NURSE-UK**)
Optionally, include the e-mail address at which you wish to receive list mail.
(eg **SUBSCRIBE [listname] [address]**)

To leave a list:

Lisproc: **UNSUBSCRIBE [listname]**

Listserv: **SIGNOFF [listname]** or **UNSUBSCRIBE [listname]**

Mailbase: **LEAVE [listname]**

Mailserv: **UNSUBSCRIBE [listname]** or **UNSUBSCRIBE [listname] [address]**
(if you subscribed under a different e-mail address)

Majordomo: **UNSUBSCRIBE [listname]** or **UNSUBSCRIBE [listname] [address]**
(if you subscribed under a different e-mail address)

To receive the list in digest format (multiple messages compiled into a single mailing, usually daily or weekly):

Listproc: **SET [listname] MAIL DIGEST**

Listserv: **SET [listname] DIGEST**

Mailbase: not supported.

Mailserv: not supported.

Majordomo: **SUBSCRIBE [listname]-DIGEST** (see below)
In the same message, unsubscribe from the undigested version (eg **UNSUBSCRIBE [listname]**)

Note: With those programs that support the digest option, whether or not to offer the digest format is within the discretion of the list owner; consequently, not all lists offer digests.

To cancel digest format and receive the list as separate mailings:

Listproc: **SET [listname] MAIL ACK**

Listserv: **SET [listname] MAIL**

Mailbase: not supported.

Mailserv: not supported.

DISPLAY 3-1. GLOSSARY OF MAIL SERVER COMMANDS (CONTINUED)

Majordomo: **UNSUBSCRIBE [listname]-DIGEST**
In the same message, subscribe to the undigested version (eg **SUBSCRIBE [listname]**)

To suspend mail temporarily (without unsubscribing):
Listproc: **SET [listname] MAIL POSTPONE**
Listserv: **SET [listname] NOMAIL**
Mailbase: **SUSPEND MAIL [listname]**
Mailserv: not supported.
Majordomo: not supported.

To resume receipt of messages:
Listproc: **SET [listname] MAIL ACK** or **SET [listname]MAIL NOACK** or **SET [listname] MAIL DIGEST**
Listserv: **SET [listname] MAIL** or **SET [listname] DIGEST**
Mailbase: **RESUME MAIL [listname]**
Mailserv: not supported.
Majordomo: not supported.

To receive copies of your own messages:
Listproc: **SET [listname] MAIL ACK**
Listserv: **SET [listname] REPRO** (To simply receive an automatic acknowledgment that your message has been sent to the list, use: **SET [listname] ACK**)
Mailbase: standard feature; you always receive your own messages.
Mailserv: same as Mailbase.
Majordomo: same as Mailbase.

To not receive copies of your own messages:
Listproc: **SET [listname] MAIL NOACK**
Listserv: **SET [listname] NOREPRO**
Mailbase: not supported.
Mailserv: not supported.
Majordomo: not supported.

To obtain a list of subscribers:
Listproc: **RECIPIENTS [listname]**
Listserv: **REVIEW [listname] F=MAIL**
Can also be sorted by name or country.
(eg **REVIEW [listname] BY NAME F=MAIL** or **REVIEW [listname] BY COUNTRY F=MAIL**)
Mailbase: **REVIEW [listname]**
Mailserv: **SEND/LIST [listname]**
Majordomo: **WHO [listname]**

(continued)

DISPLAY 3-1.   GLOSSARY OF MAIL SERVER COMMANDS (CONTINUED)

To hide your address so that it does not appear on the list of subscribers:
Listproc: **SET [listname] CONCEAL YES**
               To reverse this command, use: **SET [listname] CONCEAL NO**
Listserv: **SET [listname] CONCEAL**
               To reverse this command, use: **SET [listname] NOCONCEAL**
Mailbase: not supported.
Mailserv: not supported.
Majordomo: not supported.

To obtain a list of lists maintained by this mail server:
Listproc: **LISTS**
Listserv: **LISTS**
               To obtain a list of all known Listserv lists, send the command **LISTS
               GLOBAL.** To search for Listserv lists with a given keyword or character
               string in the description, send the command **LISTS GLOBAL /[keyword].**
               (eg **LISTS GLOBAL /NURSING**)
Mailbase: **LISTS**
Mailserv: **DIRECTORY/LIST**
Majordomo: **LISTS**

To obtain a listing of archive files for a particular list:
Listproc: **INDEX [listname]**
Listserv: **INDEX [listname]**
Mailbase: **INDEX [listname]**
Mailserv: **INDEX [listname]**
Majordomo: **INDEX [listname}**

To retrieve an archive file:
Listproc: **GET [listname] [filename]**
         (eg, **GET PERIOP feb98**)
Listserv: **GET [filename] [filetype] [listname] F=MAIL**
         (eg, **GET NURSERES LOG9806 NURSERES F=MAIL**)
Mailbase: **SEND [listname] [filename]**
         (eg, **SEND NURSE-ROGERS 05-1998**)
Mailserv: **SEND [listname] [filename]**
         (eg, **SEND PEDIATRIC-PAIN smith.txt**)
Majordomo: **GET [listname] [filename]**
         (eg, **GET NURSE-UK BOYLE.TXT**)

Adapted with permission from Hancock L. *Physician's Guide to the Internet.* Philadelphia, PA: Lippincott-
Raven, 1996, and "Discussion Lists: Mail Server Commands," prepared by James Milles, Head of Computer Services, St. Louis University Law Library, St. Louis, MO 63108; e-mail: millesjg @sluvca. slu.edu

on the mainframe computer for a period of time. Think of the difference between receiving mail and reading a bulletin board. With a Listserv, you get the mail in your mailbox and have to deal with it, even if that means simply hitting the delete key. With Usenet groups, you are reading the messages posted on a bulletin board. If you do not happen to walk by the bulletin board, you will not see the messages.

As a point of information, some Listserv discussions are also echoed to the news groups. This gives you the opportunity to choose how you get your information. For example, the Listserv STAT-L is a consultation group for statistics. It is echoed to the Usenet group sci.stat.consult. If you are a researcher, engaged in statistical analysis on a regular basis, you might appreciate the ongoing discussion of statistical procedures, problems, and solutions. On the other hand, if you are a more casual user, you might be glad to know about the sci.stat.consult group but choose to read it only when you have a specific question in mind that you would like to have answered.

Just about every topic imaginable is covered somewhere in a Usenet news group. While not technically part of the Internet, Usenet news groups are generally available through Unix computers connected to the Internet. They are like an uncensored orphan of the Internet and a great source of information and fun. Some might say that the Usenet groups are an acquired taste. There are more than 5000 topics covered, with new ones being added and outdated ones deleted daily. How long the messages stay in the system depends on the system operator; most purge old messages every few weeks.

A news reader program is used to access the messages for reading. There are many news readers, each with a different look, that are provided by Internet access providers or that come bundled in Internet software packages. Like Listserv lists, Usenet news groups are usually free to the person connected to the Internet.

Usenet groups have a specific hierarchical naming system. The names look odd at first, but the system makes sense once you get the hang of it. The first part of the name describes the general kind of news group; the next part describes the type of group more specifically, and so on. So, for example, groups that start with sci have to do with science; sci.med groups are those related to the medical sciences. The nursing discussion is located at sci.med.nursing, to many nurses' dismay. However, the naming has nothing to do with the role of nursing as related to the role of medicine, and it is not an attempt to disempower nurses. It only relates to science, then medical sciences, then nursing. A listing of the top level names of several Usenet groups is presented in Display 3-2.

If you are searching for nursing- and health-related discussions, your best bet will be to look in the sci.med groups and the alt.support groups. The former are generally discussions among health professionals; the latter include a wide range of participants, including patients, their families, and health care providers. Before you use information from a group discussion, or before you refer a patient or colleague to a discussion, be sure to check it out and satisfy yourself in

DISPLAY 3-2. TOP-LEVEL NAMES OF USENET GROUPS

alt:
Alternative groups. Setting up a group in any of the following hierarchies is an involved process, requiring a charter and online vote. Anyone can set up an alt group. Many times, after it has been around for a while, the readers will pursue having it become a mainstream group, although there are many alt groups that have been around for years and show no evidence of changing.

comp:
Topics dealing with computers.

sci:
Topics dealing with the sciences.

sci.med:
Medical- and health-related science discussions.

rec:
Recreational newsgroups, including sports, hobbies, and the arts.

soc:
Social newsgroups, including social interests and socializing.

news:
Topics having to do with Internet news itself.

talk:
Long arguments, frequently political.

your own mind that the information is indeed what you expect and need. This is important because many of your patients may find their way to some of the patient support groups. Perhaps you are a diabetes educator. While you may choose not to refer patients or clients to alt.support.diabetes, if you have computer-literate patients, they may find the group on their own. You would be wise to visit the group, follow the discussions, and assess the information so that, if you are asked about it, you can given an informed answer about the content that is available.

BEING REALISTIC: WHAT TO EXPECT ON YOUR INTERNET JOURNEY

So far, I have covered how to travel and what to see on the Internet. Are you ready to venture forth? Probably. But I want to include a few words of warning about what you can and cannot expect on your journey. I have friends who have traveled to Jamaica, expecting a tropical paradise, but have been shocked to discover the poverty that exists in that small island nation. The Internet is the same way. As you prepare for your journey, keep the following in mind.

What to Expect

The first thing to expect on your Internet journey is confusion. People have described the Internet as the modern equivalent of the Wild West frontier, and at times that seems to be an apt description. Although things are becoming more organized out there in the Internet world, a high degree of confusion still exists. Give yourself some time to learn your way around and discover how to best find the information you are seeking. Do not expect to become an expert overnight. I have been at this for several years now, and some days I still feel like a novice.

Prepare yourself for lots of irrelevant material. In discussion groups, for example, people have a way of getting off track. Although the header says, "Breast cancer research results," the message might not have anything to do with breast cancer or research. It is common to hear people discuss the "high signal-to-noise ratio" on the Internet. This simply means that for every useful bit of information you find, you'll have to sift through an equal number of useless bits.

You can also expect to find a virtual community. This is one of the pleasant surprises of the Internet. Although there are millions of people accessing the Internet every day, you'll quickly learn the names and personalities of the members of your Internet world. In particular, I have found that nurses on the Internet are a very friendly group. As a group, we tend to be quick to offer help, answer questions, share experiences, and talk about nursing. Nurses on the Internet are tolerant of newbies (those new to the Net), keep flaming to a minimum (especially compared with some of the more virulent groups), and are even accepting of NRNs.[2] Clinicians, researchers, teachers, administrators, and many nurses from around the globe form our virtual community.

The Internet is a great leveler. You are interacting with people in nontraditional ways. Issues that sometimes get in the way of traditional communication, such as gender, skin color, height, or weight, become irrelevant on the Internet. People are free to have open, honest discussions. Of course, having these discussions is a special privilege. Respect the time and information that people share with you, and do not trivialize their contributions.

Finally, things happen quickly on the Internet. You can post a question and may have several answers within minutes. Be prepared for this both in terms of receiving and responding to messages. I occasionally post requests to the nurse educators discussion group asking for software reviewers for *Computers in Nursing*. Replies have come back to me in as little as 60 seconds! I learned very quickly not to post such a request on a day when I would not be in my office and not able to check my e-mail at frequent intervals.

---

[2]NRN stands for "not an RN," that is, a person who is not a nurse. Gary Hales, founding editor of *Computers in Nursing*, is credited with coining this term.

What Not to Expect

Just as you can expect to find a wealth of useful information, there are certain things you should not expect on the Internet. Many people begin their journey with unrealistic expectations and then are disappointed when the trip does not deliver. Here are a few things to remember as you begin your journey.

YOU WILL NOT FIND FULL TEXT

In fact, that is not entirely true. You will find some full text, but not all of the items you might want in full text will be available. Nurses want full text of journal articles, nursing texts, patient education materials, and the like. For the most part, these types of materials are available in a limited way on the Internet.

There are online searching services, such as Internet GratefulMed (IGM, http://igm.nlm.nih.gov), that will allow you to search for journal citations in the MEDLINE database of the National Library of Medicine (NLM). Approximately 70% of the entries in MEDLINE include abstracts, and they can be retrieved using IGM. You can use Loansome Doc to order the articles from a cooperating library. But you cannot find the full text of articles online through MEDLINE. The National Library of Medicine has developed a new service, PUBMED, which has full text available for a limited number of articles, but there are fees associated with accessing this information. Another example is the UnCover database from CARL. Searching is free, but if you want an article, you pay for the document delivery service. A colleague recently described these systems as menus in a restaurant: they don't charge you to read the menu, but they charge you when they bring you your food.

At the Lippincott Nursing Center, it is possible to find full text of recent articles from some of its journals, such as the *American Journal of Nursing*. These are put up for a limited time and then taken down. If you do a literature search and need an older article, you will need to rely on traditional retrieval methods, such as a trip to the library or interlibrary loan.

At the site for the Agency for Health Care Policy and Research (AHCPR, http://www.ahcpr.gov/), you can search and download full text of its clinical practice guidelines. This is an example of full text that is available and is certainly a useful resource to know about. But before you immediately log on and start downloading one of the documents, such as the *Guideline for the Management of Cancer Pain*, remember this: the printed guideline, available for free from AHCPR, is a handy book, 6" × 9" in size with 245 pages. It is formatted and includes figures, tables, and an index. If you were to download and print this same document, it would be much more than 245 pages! Your printed version would be on 8½" × 11" sheets, and the volume would be large enough to fill a notebook. Each section of the guideline, including tables and figures, is in a separate file, and each must be downloaded individually. As a test, I downloaded the "WHO Analgesic Ladder," which is a figure in Chapter 1 of the guideline. Downloading the figure took slightly more than 4 minutes; printing it took about 3 minutes.

The time, effort, and resources that would be necessary to download the entire guideline should be carefully considered. A phone call to the toll-free number at AHCPR might be a better approach!

Of course, a major advantage of the online version is the ability to search the document. The online version also includes hypertext links to the references in the guideline. Both of these features are useful and unavailable in the printed version.

NOT EVERYTHING IS FREE

Remember the expression, "There is no such thing as a free lunch"? This is often true on the Internet. Although the Internet was designed from its roots to be a noncommercial service, that does not mean all Internet resources are free. You may need to pay or subscribe to obtain access to certain services. For example, HealthLinks (www.healthlinks.net) advertises itself as a specialized search service that will e-mail you when new health and medical sites are established on the Internet. To obtain this service, be prepared to pay $39.95 for a 1-year subscription.

Similarly, the *Online Journal of Knowledge Synthesis for Nursing* (http://www.oclc.org/oclc/forms/ojksn.htm) requires a subscription (currently $60 per year) for access. If you are not a subscriber, you will not be able to access the journal. While subscribing to journals in the non-Internet world is commonplace, many people are surprised when they encounter it on the Internet.

As the Internet continues to grow and mature, sites that were once free now require a fee or have a membership charge. For example, the Oncology Nurses Society (http://www.ons.org) site has very limited offerings available to non-members. Whether or not this trend will continue, only time can tell.

BECOMING AN EXPLORER

Once you have become comfortable as an Internet traveler, you'll be ready to move to the world of exploration. This guide is designed to provide a broad overview of useful health- and nursing-related resources. The sites in the Directory might be all you ever need. But if you decide to venture beyond what I have culled for you, you need to become comfortable with Internet searching and others ways of getting around.

Tips for Using Search Engines to Explore the Internet

Search engines are tools that enable you to expand from finding a single source of information (one Website) to locating several sites related to a single subject. There are many different search engines available on the Internet. By far, the most popular right now are the search engines that are available for the World

Wide Web. However, there are also search programs for specific functions, such as Veronica (for Gopher) and Archie (for FTP). No matter what engine you are using, the following tips apply for effective searching.

First, identify your search. Are you looking for broad information on cancer, or are you looking for patient education resources to recommend to breast cancer patients? Narrowing the topic of your search as much as possible will help you to search the Internet more efficiently. Know exactly what it is you are searching for before you start your search.

Choose the right search engine. There are many popular search engines, such as Alta Vista, InfoSeek, WebCrawler, and HotBot. All have features that distinguish themselves from each other. If you use Alta Vista, you can scour the Internet for the most obscure resources, but you may have to pull information out from among 10,000 other found references (called *hits*). Yahoo allows you to search using defined categories that will usually render fewer hits, but you may miss some important information. Try the same search in a variety of search engines and see what you retrieve. This is a good way to become familiar with the different engines and what they are able to offer you.

Select the key words for your search carefully. Obviously, if you are looking for breast cancer information, the words "breast" and "cancer" should be among the key words you choose. However, if those are the only words you use and you are searching with Alta Vista, you'll have 70,000 hits to pore through. To make this search more efficient, ask yourself, "Breast cancer information in relation to what?" Choosing additional key words such as "organizations," "Usenet," and "support" will help you to narrow your search to a manageable number of hits.

Learn to use the features of the search engine to narrow your search. If you need the most up-to-date information, you may define a specific time period in the search field. You may be able to use advanced query language (also called Boolean searches) such as "and," "not," and "or" to define your search. You might want to search only Websites or Usenet groups. Take advantage of these features and save yourself valuable time.

Brute Force Works Too

Search engines work very well, especially when you know exactly what you are looking for. For example, I recently wanted to find out how many people died in airplane crashes in 1996. With a focused search and careful selection of key words, I had the answer in 5 minutes. However, sometimes a search engine does not give you what you need. This generally happens when I want more general information. In this case, I often revert to the "brute force" method of Internet exploration.

To use brute force, try typing in an address and see what you get. The worst that can happen is that you will get an annoying message telling you the site cannot be found. Think of how the addresses work: most start with www and end with a domain name. Perhaps you are trying to find a school of nursing, let's say, at the University of New Hampshire, popularly known as UNH. Typing http://www.unh.edu will take you right to the university, and from there you can find the link to the Nursing Department home page. If your first guess doesn't work, try another; http://www.acs.org will take you to the American Chemical Society, but http://www.cancer.org takes you to the American Cancer Society.

Take Advantage of Links and Use the Bookmark Feature

Every single Website has links to other Websites of related interest. Take advantage of these links as the site developer has already done some of the work of finding other useful resources. Once again, combine brute force and links to get the information you need. Using breast cancer as an example, you might start at the American Cancer Society. There is lots of information right at the site, but you can also connect to the following:

- OncoLink, at the University of Pennsylvania
- National Breast Cancer Coalition
- Nysernet Breast Cancer Information Clearinghouse
- National Cancer Institute

These are just a few of the links available from the American Cancer Society. Each site you visit will have more links, and in this way the resources will keep building. I generally find this approach works well when I am less focused in the information I need. Visiting a variety of sites will open up the vistas of information available. When you find a site that has useful information, be sure to bookmark it. On more than one occasion, I have wasted time returning to a site of interest because I couldn't remember how I got there in the first place, and I neglected to add a bookmark to my list.

CHAPTER 4

■■■■■■■■■■■■■■■■■■■■■■■■■■■■■■■■■■■■■

How to Use the Index and Directory of Sites

The preceding three chapters have given you an overview of the Internet, an introduction to the tools necessary for exploration, and a summary of the sites you can expect to see. This chapter introduces you to the heart of the book: Part II, the Index, and Part III, the Directory of Sites.

ABOUT THE INDEX

You might be wondering why the Index is in the middle of the book when it is typically found at the back. I intentionally planned it that way. I believe the Index is the key to finding information in the Directory. Without the Index, the Directory is simply an alphabetical listing of sites. Although that is useful, combining the Directory with the Index will allow you to quickly locate specific information on a topic of interest.

One thing I have discovered in my Internet travels is that the name of a page or a site is not always descriptive of the content that is included. For example, Bo Graham has put together an excellent page of nursing, medical, and health resources (http://bgraham.com/nursing/).

It has many useful links, including several for oncology and cancer-related information. A name like "Bo Graham's Home Page," unfortunately, does not provide an inkling of what is included in the page. But a quick check under "cancer" in the Index would point you to Bo's Website.

In putting together the Index, I have tried to include every conceivable cross-reference of the information included in the Directory of Sites. Realizing that nurses work in a variety of settings, I have developed cross-reference categories that use nursing terminology as well as terminology from other fields, including disease categories and medical specialties.

As an example of how one Directory site was indexed, consider the entry for the American Association of Nurse Anesthetists (AANA). Clearly, this site has information on the AANA, so it was indexed under "Associations and Organizations." It also relates to the field of anesthesia, so it was indexed under that specialty. However, the site also has a useful information section that provides answers to common questions patients have about anesthesia, thus the site is indexed under "Consumer Information." This last bit of information is not obvious from the name of the site. If you were looking for specific patient education resources, the Index would point you to this information.

ABOUT THE DIRECTORY OF SITES

Once you have found an entry in the Index, you turn to the Directory of Sites. What can you expect to find there? A typical Directory entry is illustrated in Figure 4-1. The first line includes one of the following icons:

 means it is a site on the World Wide Web;

 means it is a Gopher site;

 means it is a Telnet site;

 refers to Listserv mailing list groups;

 refers to Usenet news groups; and

 means it is an FTP site.

There are very few U and F sites; the majority that are listed are from the WWW.

Following the site icon is the name of the site. This name is taken directly from the name present at the site. I have not changed names from those given by the developers. All sites in the Directory are arranged in strict alphabetical order (with the exception of the word "The," which has been deleted). Thus, Bo Graham's home page is under B, the American Association of Nurse Anesthetists is under A, and the *Computers in Nursing* home page is under C. My friend and colleague, Susan Newbold, was upset when she thought her home page was excluded from the first edition, as she wasn't listed under S or N. She found herself under H, as she has named her page "Home Page of Susan K. Newbold." For this edition, she has not renamed her site, so she is still in the aitches (H).

Type of site logo ☞
Name of the site ☞

Site address ☞

Site description ☞

Name and e-mail address of contact person ☞

W	**Webster's Fine Art of Nursing**
	http://www.katsden.com/nursing/index.html
	A very nice nursing site created by Kathi Webster, RN. The site is dedicated to her great-great grandfather, Aaron Webster, who was a nurse stationed near Washington DC during the Civil War.
	Contact: Kathi Webster, BSN, RN webster@katsden.com

FIGURE 4-1. Sample entry in the Directory of Sites.

Following the name of the site is the address. Once again, this has been taken directly from the site. For sites that have multiple pages, I have included the address of the home page or first page of the site. For Listservs, I have included the address to which you send your message to subscribe. I did not include the address of the list where you send your message to post to the group. That information will be sent to you once you are subscribed successfully to a group. A summary of mailing list commands is included in Chapter 3; this has not been repeated in the Directory.

Next is a brief description of the site. In many cases, I have used the descriptions provided by the sites themselves, embellishing when necessary. If a site has a particularly useful or unusual feature, I have included that information. Unusual features are often the keys to how the site is cross-referenced in the Index. If the site includes specific contact information, I have included that information, which may be a person's name and e-mail address or just an e-mail address. Note that I have not included mailing addresses, phone numbers, or fax numbers, although that information might be available at the site. As this is a guide to the Internet, I chose to include Internet contact information exclusively.

HOW SITES WERE SELECTED

When I put together the first edition of this book, with my friend and colleague Teena Ouellette, we faced a daunting task. There are millions of URLs on the World Wide Web alone, plus Gopher sites, FTP, Listserv groups, and Usenet discussion groups. We needed to develop some explicit criteria of what to include and what not to include in this Directory. The guidelines that helped us in the first edition have been helpful to me in this second edition as well.

First, this book is designed as a guide, not an encyclopedia. I have tried to be selective; my goal was not to include every site that had something to do with nursing and health, but to select sites that clearly provided useful information or, in some cases, links to other sites. If you are working in a particular specialty area, you may find sites related to your area of interest and expertise that are not included in this guide. On the other hand, I hope that the sites that are included point you to more specialized sites of interest. Remember my earlier suggestion to take advantage of links!

Let's use the Virtual Nursing College (http://www.langara.bc.ca/vnc/) as an example of what I am describing. This site, created by Jack Yensen in Vancouver, Canada, has links to a number of other sites, including nursing research, nursing informatics, pathology, and radiology. In visiting those links, I found the "Qual Page" section of Judy Norris' home page (http://www.ualberta.ca/~jrnorris/) to be a particularly interesting and useful resource; thus I included Judy's home page in the guide. (To be perfectly honest, I would have included Judy's site even if it didn't have a link from the Virtual Nursing College, but I am just trying to be illustrative!) On the other hand, the Division of General Internal Medicine at the University of California, San Francisco, was more medically oriented and seemed as if it would be of less interest for the majority of nurses who would be reading this book. However, for those of you interested in primary care and internal medicine, this site might be just what you are looking for. Although I did not include it in the guide, you could find it as a link from the Virtual Nursing College.

I also looked at the date when a site was last updated to determine whether or not to include it. Generally, I wanted evidence that the site was being regularly maintained and updated. Dates needed to be within the past 18 months to be included. With the rapid changes in health care and nursing, I figured that if a site developer has not updated a site for more than 18 months, that called into question the accuracy of the information included. The cut-off date was somewhat arbitrary, but I found it worked well to evaluate sites.

I tried to assess whether or not a site was a "going concern" in making the decision whether or not to include it. Schools of nursing and associations are obviously not going to disappear overnight. On the other hand, there are many individual home pages that just do not look like they are going to be around for the long haul. If I got repeated error messages in trying to visit a site or had problems with connection on an ongoing basis, that increased the likelihood that a site was not included.

I assessed sites for the usefulness of their content. Sites that are nothing more than a series of links to other sites ranked lower on my selection list, unless the links were very unusual or particularly comprehensive. Sites that included good content, as well as links, were deemed to be useful and were included in the guide.

I also evaluated the credentials of the people involved with the site and their clarity in communicating that message to others. For example, the OCD Home Page (http://fairlite.com/ocd/) is a site developed by a man with obsessive-compulsive disorder and his wife. He is very clear that he is not a medical or health professional and that the information offered at the site is not a substitute for medical treatment and care. Even so, I found the site to be of great interest and to contain many useful resources; thus I opted to include it.

I looked for a way to contact the site developers, either through e-mail or a feedback page. Site developers that are "anonymous," that is, not encouraging feedback or being forthcoming about their credentials, did not make it into the book.

Health On the Net Foundation

The Health On the Net Foundation has recently been established and has written a code of conduct for medical Websites. Some of the sites included in this book, but not all, included the HON Code logo, an indication that they are abiding by the principles of the code. I tried, as much as possible, to consider the HON Code Principles as I evaluated sites, but my primary criteria are included above. The HON Code principles are illustrated in Display 4-1. As you visit Websites, you would be wise to keep these principles in mind as you evaluate sites for their usefulness.

WHAT IS NOT INCLUDED

Taking the quality, not quantity, approach to selection, there are some useful resources that are not included in the Directory but are still available to you on the Web. The following types of sites were not included or were included in a selective manner.

Libraries

I opted not to include a listing of the many health and science libraries that are available via telnet. In my experience, most people connect to their local or regional library for card catalog searching. For more extensive resources, I recommend the National Library of Medicine, which is included in the Directory. If you need to search a specific health science library, you can generally connect to it from the associated university home page. To find these libraries, try brute force: www.name of university.edu. The name of the university might be an abbreviation (UNH) or the full name (Washington, for the University of Washington). Once you connect to the university, find the link to the library.

Hospitals

Like libraries, there are many hospital sites on the Web. Many of these sites would be useful for patients seeking care or nurses seeking employment; they

DISPLAY 4-1.   HEALTH ON THE NET FOUNDATION CODE OF CONDUCT FOR MEDICAL WEB SITES

Principle 1
Any medical advice provided and hosted on this site will only be given by medically trained and qualified professionals unless a clear statement is made that a piece of advice offered is from a non–medically qualified individual/organization.

Principle 2
The information provided on this site is designed to support, not replace, the relationship that exists between a patient/site visitor and his/her existing physician.

Principle 3
Confidentiality of data relating to individual patients and visitors to a medical Website, including their identity, is respected by this Website. The Website owners undertake to honor or exceed the legal requirements of medical information privacy that apply in the country and state where the Website and mirror sites are located.

Principle 4
Where appropriate, information contained on this site will be supported by clear references to source data and, where possible, have specific HTML links to that data.

Principle 5
Any claims relating to the benefits/performance of a specific treatment, commercial product, or service will be supported by appropriate, balanced evidence in the manner outlined in Principle 4 above.

Principle 6
The designers of this Website will seek to provide information in the clearest possible manner and provide contact addresses for visitors that seek further information or support. The Webmaster will display his/her e-mail address clearly throughout the Website.

Principle 7
Support for this website will be clearly identified, including the identities of commercial and noncommercial organizations that have contributed funding, services, or material for the site.

Principle 8
If advertising is a source of funding, it will be clearly stated. A brief description of the advertising policy adopted by the Website owners will be displayed on the site. Advertising and other promotional material will be presented to viewers in a manner and context that facilitates differentiation between it and the original material created by the institution operating the site.

Source: Health On the Net Foundation, http://www.hon.ch/HONcode/Conduct.html

have lists of staff, phone numbers, parking information, job postings, and the like. I chose not to include these many listings. If you are interested in finding a particular hospital, a good starting place is HospitalWeb (http://neuro-www.mgh.harvard.edu/hospitalweb.nclk), which has a constantly growing list of hospital Websites from around the country.

Schools of Nursing

When I wrote the first edition of this book, I included about 53 sites for schools and colleges of nursing. That was pretty much the universe of nursing school and college Websites at that time. Since then, there has been an explosion of sites. Many of them, however, are nothing more than the catalog put online. Although that might be a very useful resource for current and prospective students, I didn't think it would be terribly helpful for my readers. Thus, I have included only those school and college sites that had something above and beyond the program description and faculty roster. I have identified these extras in the Directory.

If you are interested in finding a particular school or college to learn more about the program, visit the National Institute of Nursing Research (http://www.nih.gov/ninr/) or Nursing-HealthWeb (http://www.lib.umich.edu/hw/nursing.html). Both have comprehensive lists of nursing programs. And if the program you want is not on one of those lists, try brute force—it really works!

Government Listings

Although I included many federal government agencies, I did not include listings of each state government Website. A good list can be found at AORN Online (http://www.aorn.org) in the legislative section.

THE PERSONAL TOUCH

To select sites, I visited each and every Website listed in the Directory, some several times. I telenetted to the telnet sites and FTPed to the FTP sites. I subscribed to every Listserv included to verify the address and purpose. For the descriptions, I relied on what the list returned to me as an introduction. If you subscribe and the discussion is not what you expected, it is easy enough to unsubscribe.

Finally, I tried as much as possible to be objective, but this Internet business is fraught with subjectivity. If it weren't, how could sites like "Worst of the Web"[1]

---

[1]Worst of the Web can be found at http://www.worstoftheweb.com/

and "Cool Site of the Day"[2] continue to exist? My personal biases and areas of interest will probably show through here and there in sites and descriptions, but my goal was to be as broad based as possible. My experience in nursing, public policy, and management, as well as my experience serving as Editor-in-Chief of *Computers in Nursing*, contributed to the overall selection process.

To this end, I would appreciate your feedback. If there are particular sites you like that I have not included, please send me the information. Many of the sites included in this second edition came directly from readers' suggestions. My e-mail address is LNICOLL@maine.maine.edu or LeslieN@muskie2.usm.maine. edu. There are also links to my address at the *Computers in Nursing* home page (http://www.cini.com/cin/) for you to communicate with me directly. If there is a site you feel would be a useful addition to this book, send it to me along with the complete address and a brief description. Similarly, if there are sites that are included that are no longer active or just not useful, please let me know that too. I consider this guide to be a work in progress and will be updating it with information that I receive from readers. I look forward to hearing from you.

As I noted earlier, an informed traveler is an intelligent traveler. Take a few minutes to familiarize yourself with the information contained in Parts II and III. And then you'll be ready to begin your journey.

---

[2]Cool Site of the Day can be found at http://cool.infi.net/

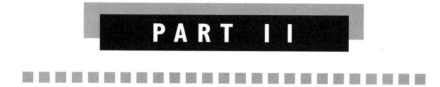

PART II

INDEX

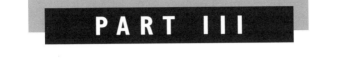

PART III

DIRECTORY OF SITES

L AANURSES

AANURSES@ontosystems.com

Discussion group for nurses and other health care professionals in recovery from alcoholism, drug addiction, eating disorders, gambling, codependency, and other obsessive-compulsive disease. This list is confidential, and requests to join will be screened by the list owner.

Type the word "subscribe" (no quotes) in the message line.

W Aboriginal Nurses Association of Canada

http://www.anac.on.ca/

Welcome to the Aboriginal Nurses Association of Canada online! ANAC is a nongovernmental, nonprofit organization whose membership works mainly in First Nations Communities. An affiliate group of the Canadian Nurses Association, it is the only Aboriginal professional nursing organization in Canada.

Contact: info@anac.on.ca

W Academic Journal Directory–University of Texas

http://www.son.utmb.edu/catalog/catalog.htm

Welcome to the online version of the University of Texas School of Nursing at Galveston's Academic Journal Directory. This document is provided as a service to the nursing and professional health care community. The directory contains listings for approximately 400 professional academic journals in clinical nursing, nursing education, nursing research, and related health care fields. A typical entry contains the full name of the journal; its publisher; its frequency of publication; its intended readership; the types of manuscripts it reviews; and a statement of purpose or general submission guidelines for prospective authors, or both. A contact address for each journal is included as well. The directory is organized alphabetically as well as by subject area.

Contact: Lara Duhon, lduhon@sonpo.utmb.edu

⌊L⌋ ACHNE-L

listserv@unccvm.uncc.edu

Discussion list for the Association of Community Health Nursing Educators.

Subscribe ACHNE-L Firstname Lastname

⟨W⟩ ACOR–Association of Cancer Online Resources

http://www.acor.org/

ACOR is a starting point for a variety of online resources related to cancer. A particularly useful feature is the Cancer Archives, a searchable database of most of the existing cancer-related news lists on the Net. Cancer Archives is a "living medical encyclopedia" wherein visitors can search the archives and indexes of cancer Listservs covering brain, hematologic, breast, ovarian, and prostate cancer.

⌊L⌋ ADDCTNSG

listproc@list.ab.umd.edu

Discussion list for the scholarly, academic, and clinical issues related to the practice of addictions nursing.

Subscribe ADDCTNSG Firstname Lastname

⟨W⟩ Addison-Wesley Nursing Network

http://heg-school.awl.com/awnrsng/awnrsng.htm

"Thank you for visiting Addison-Wesley Nursing Network, leading publisher of nursing textbooks and other learning materials. Browse our entire catalog online. Explore exercises, case studies, and quizzes on a variety of topics in the Virtual Nursing Classroom. Find out how to conduct an online job search and explore potential consulting opportunities in Resources for Nurses."

Contact: feedback@awl.com

ADDULT

listserv@maelstrom.stjohns.edu

Discussion group for adults with attention-deficit disorder.

Subscribe ADDULT Firstname Lastname

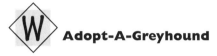

http://www.adopt-a-greyhound.org

Home page of the Greyhound Project, Inc., with information on greyhound adoption and rescue. Good resources for greyhounds as family pets.

W **Agency for Health Care Policy and Research (AHCPR)**

http://www.ahcpr.gov/

The AHCPR home page has links to its 14 offices and centers, news and resources, the Research Activities online newsletter, data and methods information, clinical practice guidelines, an electronic catalog, a search function, and other useful resources. They are regularly adding many new features. The site includes a link to the Department of Health and Human Services.

Contact: info@ahcpr.gov

 AGING-DD

listserv@ukcc.uky.edu

Aging-DD is an open forum that welcomes discussion, information, and materials on aging and older persons with developmental disabilities.

Subscribe AGING-DD Firstname Lastname

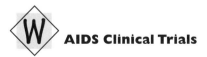

http://www.critpath.org/trials.htm

This site features the full texts of the open protocols of the major clinical trials networks. You may also peruse guides to entering clinical trials and evaluating them, expanded access programs, buyers' clubs, and patient assistance programs.

Contact: kiyoshi@critpath.org

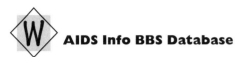 **AIDS Info BBS Database**

http://aidsinfobbs.org/

Here is a treasure house of information about AIDS. It has been building since 1985, always selecting the best but never accumulating the most. You will find that much of your selection work has already been done for you before you begin reading here. On controversial points, this collection presents both sides of the major issues, clearly labeled so you can avoid them if desired.

Contact: Ben Gardiner, ben@aidsinfobbs.org

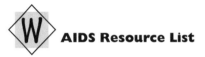 **AIDS Resource List**

http://www.teleport.com/~celinec/aids.shtml

This page offers annotated links to AIDS-related Websites, Gophers, and Usenets throughout the world. Visitors here are also invited to show support for preventing the spread of HIV and for those with the disease by downloading a small red ribbon from this home page and placing it on their own Web pages.

Contact: celinec@teleport.com

 ALLERGY

Listserve@listserv.tamu.edu

A discussion group on allergies, for allergy sufferers and health professionals.

Subscribe ALLERGY Firstname Lastname

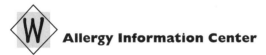 **Allergy Information Center**

http://www.kww.com/allergy/

This Website is being provided as a public service to all allergy sufferers so they can get more information about allergies, what causes them, how to live with them, and what they can do to eliminate them or get relief.

Contact: allergy@kww.com

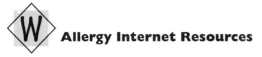

Allergy Internet Resources

http://www.io.com/~kinnaman/allabc.html

An index to documents and sites on the Internet with information about allergies of all kinds. The index is divided into the following categories: General Information; Asthma; Food Allergies; Kids' Allergies; Latex Allergy; Hay Fever, Airborne, and Seasonal Allergies; Skin Allergies; and Stings, Testing, and Anaphylaxis. A link at the bottom of the index will take you to information about the allergy e-mail discussion group, complete with an archive of recent postings to the group.

Contact: Allergylinks@immune.com

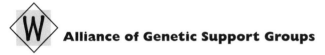

Alliance of Genetic Support Groups

http://medhlp.netusa.net/www/agsg.htm

The Alliance of Genetic Support Groups is a nonprofit organization dedicated to helping individuals and families who have genetic disorders. Their toll-free helpline is a resource for consumers and professionals who are looking for genetic support groups and genetic services. Main subject headings include Membership Application, List of Publications, Events, and Directory of National Genetic Voluntary Organizations.

Contact: alliance@capaccess.org

ALT.SUPPORT

The Usenet groups that start with "alt.support" tend to be discussions among patients, families, and interested persons including health professionals about diseases, health problems, disabilities, and the like. Some of the alt.support Usenet groups cover abortion, AIDS, arthritis, asthma, breastfeeding, cancer, cerebral palsy, chronic pain, depression, diabetes, endometriosis, epilepsy, glaucoma, hemophilia, herpes, menopause, multiple sclerosis, obsessive-compulsive disorder, ostomy, post-polio syndrome, schizophrenia, sleep disorders, thyroid disease, tinnitus, and post-traumatic stress disorder.

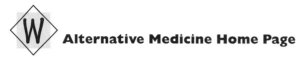
Alternative Medicine Home Page

http://www.pitt.edu/~cbw/altm.html

Maintained by the Falk Library for the Health Sciences at the University of Pittsburgh, this page is a jump station for sources of information on unconventional, unorthodox, unproven, or alternative, complementary, innovative, integrative therapies.

Contact: Charles B. Wessel, cbw@med.pitt.edu

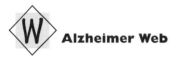
Alzheimer Web

http://dsmallpc2.path.unimelb.edu.au/ad.html

A resource for Alzheimer's disease researchers and for the people who have an interest in research developments. The home page includes news, articles, job opportunities, grants, and conference reports.

Contact: David Small, d.small@pathology.unimelb.edu.au

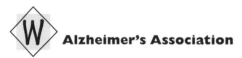
Alzheimer's Association

http://www.alz.org/

Visitors can find the Alzheimer's Association mission statement here as well as a recent archive of media releases and position statements. Medical researchers interested in funding for research on Alzheimer's disease will find information about research grants programs. There is also a listing of 200 chapter locations, caregiver resources, medical information, conferences and events, and links to other Alzheimer's Web pages.

Contact: webmaster@alz.org

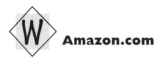
Amazon.com

http://www.amazon.com

"The Earth's Biggest Bookstore" with 2.5 million titles. Secure online ordering and speedy delivery. You can buy nursing books here, many at a discount.

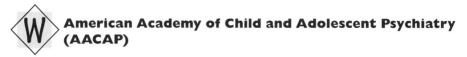

American Academy of Child and Adolescent Psychiatry (AACAP)

http://www.aacap.org/

Home page of the AACAP. A particularly useful component of this page is a collection of 56 "Facts for Families," fact sheets on various problems of childhood and adolescence. The sheets are available in English, French, and Spanish and may be downloaded, copied, and distributed as needed.

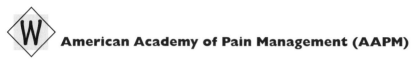

American Academy of Pain Management (AAPM)

http://www.aapainmanage.org/index.html

Site for the home page of the American Academy of Pain Management (AAPM). AAPM is the largest multidisciplinary pain society and the largest physician-based pain society in the United States. The site includes information on the organization and membership and a variety of patient resources. It is also possible to access the National Pain Databank, with live data on treatments and outcomes for specific conditions for more than 9,500 patients.

Contact: aapm@aapainmanage.org

American Academy of Pediatrics (AAP)

http://www.aap.org/

A voice for children for more than 60 years, the American Academy of Pediatrics (AAP) is an organization of 50,000 pediatricians dedicated to the health, safety, and well-being of infants, children, adolescents, and young adults. The AAP Website has news, membership information, other child health resources, and information for parents and health professionals.

Contact: kidsdocs@aap.org or webmaster@aap.org

American Association for the History of Nursing (AAHN)

http://users.aol.com/nsghistory/AAHN.html

The American Association for the History of Nursing (AAHN) is a professional organization open to everyone interested in the history of nursing. Originally founded in 1978 as a historical methodology group, the association was briefly named the International History of Nursing Society. The organization's purposes are to stimulate national and international interest in the history of nursing, promote collaboration among its supporters, encourage research in the history of nursing, promote the development of centers for the preservation and use of materials of historical importance to nursing, serve as a resource for information related to nursing history, and produce and distribute materials related to the history and heritage of the nursing profession.

Contact: Janet L. Fickeissen, NsgHistory@aol.com

W   American Association for Therapeutic Humor

http://ideanurse.com/aath/

Working at a frenzied pace in a hospital or doctor's office would be enough to wear down anyone's funny bone. As a counterbalance, the American Association for Therapeutic Humor was created to help health professionals maintain a sense of humor about the world around them. The AATH Website features a collection of articles from the therapeutic humor literature, plus a collection of "Twelve Affirmations of Positive Humor" and links to other therapeutic humor Websites, such as the *Journal of Nursing Jocularity.*

W   American Association of Colleges of Nursing

http://www.aacn.nche.edu/

Home page of AACN, the national voice for America's baccalaureate- and higher-degree nursing education programs.

Contact: webmaster@aacn.nche.edu.

W   American Association of Critical-Care Nurses

http://www.aacn.org/

The American Association of Critical-Care Nurses was founded in 1969 and now, almost 30 years later, has grown to become the world's largest specialty nursing organization with more than 76,000 members around the world. The vision of AACN is a health care system, driven by the needs of patients, where critical care nurses make their optimal contribution. This site has information on certification, publications, a calendar of events, an online catalog, a list of association chapters, and membership information.

Contact: info@aacn.org

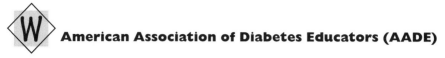

American Association of Diabetes Educators (AADE)

http://www.diabetesnet.com/aade.html

AADE is made up of a wide variety of health professionals who are involved in educating people with diabetes. AADE has a number of state and regional chapters, puts on educational conferences for health professionals, and is a great source (via the Diabetes Educator Access Line) for referrals to nurse educators and physicians in your area who specialize in diabetes. The organization sponsors the C.D.E. certification program for diabetes educators. It also provides some grants, scholarships, and awards for educational research and teaching activities.

American Association of Legal Nurse Consultants

http://www.aalnc.org/

The American Association of Legal Nurse Consultants (AALNC) is a nonprofit organization dedicated to the professional enhancement of registered nurses practicing in a consulting capacity in the legal field. Founded in 1989, AALNC serves as a resource for its members by providing opportunities for continuing education and an exchange of information on matters relating to legal nurse consulting, medical care, and health care law.

Contact: webmaster@aalnc.org

American Association of Neuroscience Nurses (AANN)

http://www.aann.org

The American Association of Neuroscience Nurses is a specialty organization serving nurses throughout the world. More than 4000 career-minded nurses in the United States and a dozen foreign countries belong to the AANN for the networking and continuing education it provides. The AANN Web page has links to news, FAQs, an events calendar, and other chapters. There are also pointers to the Neuroscience Nursing Foundation and the *Journal of Neuroscience Nursing.*

Contact: AssnNeuro@aol.com

American Association of Nurse Anesthetists (AANA)

http://www.aana.com/

The AANA Website has major headings of patient resources, member resources, and professional resources. Patients can access related information describing anesthesia and its affects and their role in the recovery process. Members can find organizational information such as contacts, events, educational offerings, and anesthesia-related Web resources. Professional resources include information on history, legal issues, cost-effectiveness of nurse anesthesia practice, and educational opportunities.

American Association of Occupational Health Nurses

http://www.aaohn.org/

This is the home page of the AAOHN, whose mission is to advance the profession of occupational and environmental health nursing.

American Cancer Society

http://www.cancer.org/

The American Cancer Society home page has information on their organization and local chapters, cancer information, a calendar of events, publications, and resources. There are also pointers to the Relay for Life, the Breast Cancer Network, the Great American SmokeScream, and Comprehensive School Health Education.

American College of Nurse Midwives (ACNM)

http://www.acnm.org/

The mission of ACNM is to develop and support the profession to promote the health and well-being of women and infants within their families and communities. The philosophy inherent in the profession states that nurse-midwives believe every individual has the right to safe, satisfying health care with respect for human dignity and cultural variations. The ACNM page has information on how to find nurse-midwives, nurse-midwifery education and certification,

ACNM and midwifery information, ACNM chapter information, and other nursing resources.

Contact: info@acnm.org

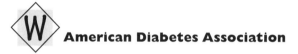

American College of Nurse Practitioners

http://www.nurse.org/acnp/

Home page of the American College of Nurse Practitioners.

Contact: acnp@nurse.org

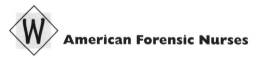

American Diabetes Association

http://www.diabetes.org/professional.htm

The mission of the American Diabetes Association is "to prevent and cure diabetes, and to improve the lives of all people affected by diabetes." To fulfill this mission, the American Diabetes Association funds research; publishes scientific findings; and provides information and other services to people with diabetes, their families, health care professionals, and the public. This home page has the latest news on diabetes, a message from the leadership, and an information directory. Visitors can also find contact information for local offices.

Contact: klowe@diabetes.org

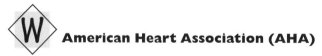

American Forensic Nurses

http://www.amrn.com/

Information on American Forensic Nurses, their work, and their goals. Distance courses that can be taken via the WWW are available at this site.

American Heart Association (AHA)

http://www.amhrt.org/

The AHA Web page contains information about the organization, patient information, support group links, licensed products and services, and science and research. There are also pointers to other heart and cardiovascular servers maintained by government agencies and nongovernment societies and associations.

Contact: inquire@amhrt.org

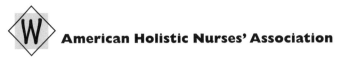

American Holistic Nurses' Association

http://www.ahna.org/

Home page of the AHNA, this site contains information on the association, education, certification, and standards for holistic nursing. Find out about the Nightingale Moment (May 12, 2000) at this site.

Contact: webmaster@ahna.org

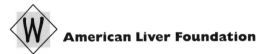

American Liver Foundation

http://sadieo.ucsf.edu/alf/alffinal/

Home page of the American Liver Foundation, the only national, voluntary nonprofit health agency dedicated to preventing, treating, and curing hepatitis and all liver diseases through research, education, and support groups. Site includes information for physicians, nurses, other health professionals, patients, and their families.

Contact: webmail@liverfoundation.org

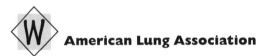

American Lung Association

http://www.lungusa.org/index.html

"When you can't breathe, nothing else matters." Good, informative site on respiratory and related illnesses. Be sure to check out the Phlemmy Awards!

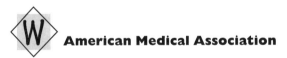

American Medical Association

http://www.ama-assn.org/

Home page of the AMA. This site includes full text of selected articles from their journals, including *JAMA*, news releases, and abstracts. There are information centers on migraine, asthma, HIV, and kids health. The On-Line Doctor Finder is a handy resource for patients and professionals.

Contact: WebAdmin@ama-assn.org

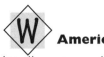 **American Nurses Association**

http://www.ana.org/ or http://www.nursingworld.org

Home page of the ANA with links to state organizations, legislative issues, and membership information. This site is also the home of the American Academy of Nursing, American Nurses Credentialing Center, American Nurses Foundation, and the Ethnic Minority Fellowship Project. The *Online Journal of Issues in Nursing* (see separate listing for OJIN) can also be accessed at this site.

Contact: webfeedback@ana.org

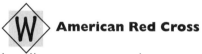 **American Physiological Society**

gopher://gopher.uth.tmc.edu:3300/1

The American Physiological Society is devoted to fostering scientific research (with special emphasis on studying the ways the body functions), education, and the dissemination of scientific information. Through its activities, it plays an important role in the progress of science and the advancement of knowledge. Some of its Gopher menu entries detail the society's structure, functions, public affairs activities, and publication programs.

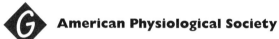 **American Red Cross**

http://www.crossnet.org/

A public relations platform for the American Red Cross, this site is maintained by the national headquarters. The mission, goals, history, financial structure, and health and safety programs of the national arm of this humanitarian organization are fully detailed. Of particular interest are the current press releases that detail relief efforts in disaster areas. A nice image map helps you locate the nearest Red Cross chapter by region or zip code.

Contact: internet@usa.redcross.org

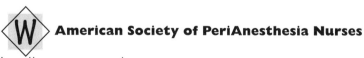 **American Society of PeriAnesthesia Nurses**

http://www.aspan.org/

Here is the home page of ASPAN, with membership information and resources relating to perianesthesia nursing.

Contact: aspan@slackinc.com

W Americans With Disabilities Act Document Center

http://janweb.icdi.wvu.edu/kinder/

This Website contains copies of the Americans With Disabilities Act of 1990 (ADA), ADA regulations, technical assistance manuals prepared by the United States Equal Employment Opportunity Commission (EEOC) or the United States Department of Justice (DOJ), and other technical assistance documents sponsored by the National Institute on Disability and Rehabilitation Research (NIDRR) and reviewed by EEOC or DOJ. There are also links to other Internet sources of information concerning disability issues, legal issues, occupational health and safety, and total quality management issues. Visitors searching for an item not found on this site can use the Internet search tools and links to libraries that this site provides. Visitors can also find information and links for the Job Accommodation Network (JAN).

Contact: Duncan Kinder, dckinder@ovnet.com

W AMIA Nursing Informatics Working Group

http://www.gl.umbc.edu/~abbott/nurseinfo.html

The overall goal of AMIA's Nursing Informatics Working Group is to promote the advancement of nursing informatics within the larger multidisciplinary context of health informatics. The organization and its members pursue this goal in many arenas: professional practice, education, research, governmental and other service, professional organizations, and industry.

Contact: Patricia A. Abbott, abbott@gl.umbc.edu

L AMPUTEE

listserv@sjuvm.stjohns.edu

Discussion group for amputees, friends, families, and health professionals.

Subscribe AMPUTEE Firstname Lastname

ANEST-L

listserv@listserv.acsu.buffalo.edu

Discussion group for anesthesiologists, nurse anesthetists, and others interested in anesthesiology and critical care.

Subscribe ANEST-L Firstname Lastname

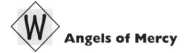 **Angels of Mercy**

http://www.aofm.com/

Resources and information for nurses, with an emphasis on home health care.

Contact: dennis@statmail.com

 ANI-L

listserv@utkvm1.utk.edu

Discussion group for Autism International Network.

Subscribe ANI-L Firstname Lastname

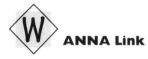 **ANNA Link**

http://www.inurse.com/~anna/

Official Website of the American Nephrology Nurses Association.

Contact: webmaster@inurse.com

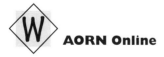 **AORN Online**

http://www.aorn.org/

Visitors to AORN Online can obtain information on the Association of Operating Room Nurses, Inc., (AORN) and its activities. There are pointers to organizational information, products and services, clinical practice information, education, government affairs, online perioperative employment opportunities, certification, and industry connections. This site also includes the "Surgery Center: A Patient's Place," a resource of patient-centered information specifically relating to surgery and the surgical process. There is a feedback form for visitor input and general membership information for AORN.

Contact: Kathryn White, webmaster@aorn.org

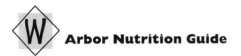

Arbor Nutrition Guide

http://arborcom.com/

A site of more than 1,000 nutrition resources. Easily searchable and well organized.

Contact: Tony Helman, helmant@ozemail.com.au

Arkansas State University College of Nursing and Health Professions

http://www.astate.edu/

This site has information on the College of Nursing and its programs. There is a useful link to the Delta Health Education Partnership from this site.

Contact: Nancy Murray, nmurray@crow.astate.edu

ARL Directory of Electronic Journals, Newsletters, and Academic Discussion Lists

gopher://arl.cni.org

Maintained by the Association of Research Libraries, this is a comprehensive list of electronic journals (e-journals), newsletters, and academic discussion groups (not just biomedical). Announcements of new e-journals are posted to the following list: NewJour-L@e-math.ams.org.

Contact: Dru Mogge, dru@cni.org

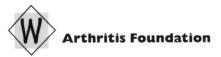

Arthritis Foundation

http://www.arthritis.org/

The mission of the Arthritis Foundation is to support research to find the cure for and prevention of arthritis, and to improve the quality of life for those affected by arthritis. Visitors to the Arthritis Foundation Web page will find news updates, fact sheets, research resources, and chapter locations. There are also links to other organizations devoted to fighting arthritis in adults and children.

Contact: webmaster@arthritis.org.

Association of Rehabilitation Nurses

http://www.rehabnurse.org//

Home page for the ARN. The site includes membership information; continuing education opportunities; news; periodicals; information on certification, grants, and scholarships; and general information for the public.

Contact: info@rehabnurse.org

Association of Women's Health, Obstetric and Neonatal Nursing

http://www.awhonn.org/

Official Website of AWHONN, whose mission is to promote excellence in nursing practice to improve the health of women and newborns. This site provides information on the organization and a wide variety of resources for obstetrical, neonatal, and women's health care.

Contact: janac@awhonn.org

Australian Electronic Journal of Nursing Education

http://www.csu.edu.au/faculty/health/nurshealth/aejne/aejnehp.htm

The *AEJNE* is committed to enhancing the teaching and learning experience across a variety of nurse contexts. The journal is a means by which nurses can share findings, insights, experience, and advice with colleagues involved in all aspects of the educational process. The *AEJNE* seeks to use the advantages of electronic communication to provide rapid and accessible information about teaching and learning to nurses worldwide. The *AEJNE* has a special commitment to nursing education in Australia. To this end, it will allow country-specific comment in this context. The universality of teaching and learning will, however, provide wide opportunity for nurses outside Australia to publish studies and papers in the journal. The editor is Peter Cleasby, (pcleasby@csu.edu.au).

Contact: aejne@csu.edu.au

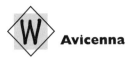

Avicenna

http://www.avicenna.com

A comprehensive medical information resource free to all health care professionals, Avicenna offers searchable databases, including free MEDLINE access, reference materials, and tools for medical practice. Registration is required, but it is free.

Contact: webmaster@avicenna.com

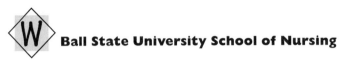

Ball State University School of Nursing

http://www.nursing.bsu.edu/

This school's home page allows the visitor to access general information, academic program and course information, and continuing education opportunities and to take a virtual tour of the Health Care Learning Resource Center.

Contact: Kay Hodson, 00kehodson@bsuvc.bsu.edu

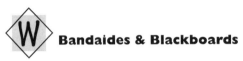

Bandaides & Blackboards

http://funrsc.fairfield.edu/~jfleitas/contents.html

This is a site about growing up with medical problems. Its goal is to help people understand what it's like, from the perspective of the children and teens who are doing just that. These kids have become experts at coping with problems that most children have never heard of. They'd like you to know how they do it, and they hope that you'll be glad you came to visit. The site is divided into three areas: one for kids, one for teens, and one for adults. Lots of useful information and some moving stories and poems can be found here.

Contact: Joan Fleitas, fleitas@fair1.fairfield.edu

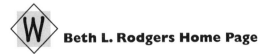

Beth L. Rodgers Home Page

http://www.uwm.edu:80/People/brodg/

Beth Rodgers is a faculty member at the University of WI–Milwaukee in the school of nursing. This page provides easy access to starting points for Internet, WWW, and computer-related information; to nursing and health-related sites;

and to some of Beth's favorite philosophy and research-related sites. As an associate editor for the international journal *Health Care in Later Life,* she has included the guidelines for authors here as well.

Contact: Beth Rodgers, brodg@csd.uwm.edu

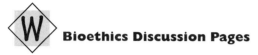

Bioethics Discussion Pages

http://www-hsc.usc.edu/~mbernste/

This site includes ongoing discussions on a variety of ethical issues. Everyone is invited to join in the discussion regarding these issues. Current topics include physician-assisted suicide, cloning, pharmaceutical testing, and life support for death row inmates.

Contact: Maurice Bernstein, MD, DoktorMo@aol.com

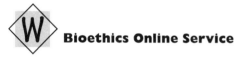

Bioethics Online Service

http://www.mcw.edu/bioethics/index.html

The Bioethics Online Service is a searchable database of abstracts of pertinent bioethics journal articles, legislative actions, and court decisions. It is maintained by the Center for the Study of Bioethics and the Office of Research, Technology, and Information of the Medical College of Wisconsin. The database is updated weekly.

Contact: Arthur R. Derse, aderse@its.mcw.edu

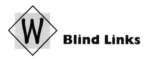

Blind Links

http://www.seidata.com/~marriage/rblind.html

A large collection of links to Internet sites related to blindness, compiled by Ron Marriage. Among the resources listed in the collection are Raised Dot Computing, the Interactive ASL and Braille Guide, and the American Foundation for the Blind server.

Contact: Ron Marriage, marriage@seidata.com

BLIND-L

listserv@uafsysb.uark.edu

Discussion group about blindness and related issues.

Subscribe BLIND-L Firstname Lastname

 ## BLINDNWS

listserv@vm1.nodak.edu

An electronic journal, *Blind News Digest,* related to blindness.

Subscribe BLINDNWS Firstname Lastname

 ## BMT TALK

listserv@listserv.acor.org

Discussion group about bone marrow transplant and related issues.

Subscribe BMT-TALK Firstname Lastname

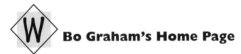 ## Bo Graham's Home Page

http://bgraham.com/nursing/

Bo Graham's pioneering home page. Although it is primarily a links page, there are many useful connections, especially related to cancer.

Contact: Bo Graham, bgraham@bgraham.com

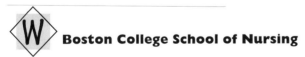 ## Boston College School of Nursing

http://www.bc.edu/bc_org/avp/son/default.html

A stop here offers information on the undergraduate, master's, and PhD programs; faculty; and scholarships. There are also links to the Center for Nursing Research, the Nursing Ethics Network, continuing education programs, Alpha Chi chapter of Sigma Theta Tau, and other nursing Websites.

Contact: Cathy Toran, toranca@bc.edu

BRAINTMR

listserv@mitvma.mit.edu

Discussion group for brain tumor patients, their families, and health professionals.

Subscribe BRAINTMR Firstname Lastname

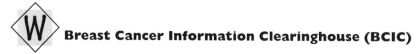

http://nysernet.org/bcic

Developed and maintained by the New York State Education and Research Network, this Website provides information on breast cancer for patients, their families, and health professionals. There is information on breast cancer detection, medical information, and support. BCIC also has links to Gophers, Listservs, and other online cancer resources.

Contact: Terri Damon, tmdamon@nysernet.org

 BREAST-CANCER

listserv@morgan.ucs.mun.ca

Discussion group on breast cancer for patients, families, and health professionals.

Subscribe BREAST-CANCER Firstname Lastname

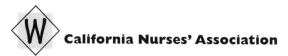

http://www.igc.apc.org/cna/

The California Nurses' Association is working together with patients and health care consumers to ensure access to safe, quality health care. CNA's Web page also contains membership and job information.

Contact: patientwatch@igc.org

CampRN

listproc@listproc.wsu.edu

Discussion list for camp nurses, camp health professionals, and camp administrators to share information, resources, ideas, and experiences about camp health care.

Subscribe CampRN Firstname Lastname

W Canadian Association of Critical Care Nurses

http://www.execulink.com/~caccn/

Home page of the Canadian Association of Critical Care Nurses with information on membership, education, and research.

W Canadian Association of Nurses in Independent Practice

http://www.websmart.com/canip/

Home page of CANIP, designed to provide a forum in which the entrepreneurial nurse may network, lobby for changes in the health care system, and receive practical and moral support in a community of nurses.

Contact: mhogg@freespace.net

W Canadian Intravenous Nurses Association

http://web.idirect.com/~csotcina/cina.html

Home page of the Canadian Intravenous Nurses Association, which is an association that unites all nurses initiating and maintaining IVs.

W Canadian Nurses Association

http://www.cna-nurses.ca/

Home page of the Canadian Nurses Association. The site is available in both English and French.

Contact: cna@cna-nurses.ca

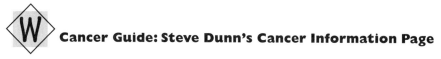

Cancer Guide: Steve Dunn's Cancer Information Page

http://cancerguide.org/

A guide for cancer patients who want to understand more about the disease and their treatment options. The author is a cancer survivor himself.

Contact: Steve Dunn, dunns@h2net.net

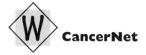

CancerNet

http://cancernet.nci.nih.gov/

Maintained by the National Cancer Institute at the National Institutes of Health, this site contains accurate, credible, cancer information. All information located on CancerNet has been reviewed by oncology experts and is based on the results of current research.

CANCER-L

listserv@wvnvm.wvnet.edu

Discussion group on cancer and related issues.

Subscribe CANCER-L Firstname Lastname

CARENET

listserv@sco.georcoll.on.ca

International discussion group to explore issues of relevance to the development of Caring Theory and its application to nursing and nursing education.

Subscribe CARENET Firstname Lastname

CARENETL

listserv@admin.humberc.on.ca

Discussion group for nurse faculty.

Subscribe CARENETL Firstname Lastname

L   CATHAR-M

listserv@maelstrom.stjohns.edu

Electronically distributed newsmagazine for chronic fatigue syndrome.

Subscribe CATHAR-M Firstname Lastname

W   Catholic University of America School of Nursing

http://www.cua.edu/www/nurs/welcome.htm

Comprehensive home page for the school of nursing, with courses, faculty, and resources. There is an interesting listing of faculty and alumni accomplishments.

Contact: cua-nursing@cua.edu

W   CCRN Net

http://www.ccrnnet.com/

Web page of Steven E. Marshall, RN, CCRN. Lots of links, especially related to critical care.

Contact: Steven E. Marshall, webmaster@ccrnnet.com

W   Center for Food Safety and Applied Nutrition

http://vm.cfsan.fda.gov/list.html

The Center for Food Safety and Applied Nutrition (CFSAN) is a department of the FDA whose mission is "to promote and protect the public health and economic interest by ensuring that the food supply is safe, nutritious, wholesome, and honest, and that cosmetics are safe and properly labeled." The CFSAN WWW site provides access to a variety of FDA publications, covering such areas as food additives, biotechnology, food labeling, and food-borne illnesses.

Contact: Larry Dusold, lrd@cfsan.fda.gov

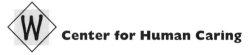 **Center for Human Caring**

http://www.uchsc.edu/ctrsinst/chc/index.htm

This page is a collection of resources for those interested in the Center for Human Caring activities and Watson's Theory of Human Caring.

Contact: Karen Holland, Karen.Holland@UCHSC.Edu

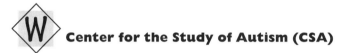 **Center for Narcolepsy Research**

http://www.uic.edu/depts/cnr/cindex.htm

Information about the Center for Narcolepsy Research, based at the College of Nursing at the University of Illinois in Chicago. Has good links to other sleep resources.

Contact: Thomas Kotsos, tkotso1@uic.edu

Center for the Study of Autism (CSA)

http://www.autism.org/

The Center for the Study of Autism (CSA) is located in the Portland, Oregon, area. Established in 1991, the center provides information about autism to parents and professionals and conducts research on the efficacy of various therapeutic interventions. Most of the research is in collaboration with the Autism Research Institute in San Diego, California. This page has links to detailed information on autism and related disorders, issues, and interventions. Basic information on autism is included in English, Chinese, Spanish, and Korean.

Contact: samr7@netcom.com

Center for the Study of the History of Nursing

http://www.upenn.edu/nursing/facres_history.html

The Center for the Study of the History of Nursing was established in 1985 to encourage and facilitate historical scholarship on health care history and nursing in the United States. Now in its 13th year, the center continues to create and maintain a resource for such research, to improve the quality and scope of historical scholarship on nursing, and to disseminate new knowledge on nursing history through education, conferences, publications, and interdisciplinary collaboration.

Contact: nhistory@pobox.upenn.edu

W Centers for Disease Control and Prevention (CDC)

http://www.cdc.gov/

CDC offers links to all of its centers, offices, and institutes; a calendar of events; and pointers to topics such as diseases, health risks, prevention guidelines and strategies, the *Morbidity and Mortality Weekly Report,* scientific data, health statistics, publications, and products.

Contact: netinfo@cdc.gov

W CenterWatch Clinical Trials Listing Service

http://www.centerwatch.com/

You can use this listing to search for clinical trials, to find out information about physicians and medical centers performing clinical research, and to learn about drug therapies newly approved by the Food and Drug Administration. You may also sign up for the e-mail notification service, which will inform you of future postings in a particular therapeutic area.

Contact: cntrwatch@aol.com

W ceWEB

http://www.ce-web.com/

Online continuing education (CE), brought to you by American Health Consultants, publishers of *Hospital Infection Control.* Topics covered include Quality/ Patient Management, Infection Control, and Outpatient and Home Health. There is a charge to take the tests and receive CE credit.

CFS-L

listserv@maelstrom.stjohns.edu

Discussion group on chronic fatigue syndrome for patients and nonhealth professionals.

Subscribe CFS-L Firstname Lastname

L **CFS-MED**

listserv@maelstrom.stjohns.edu

Discussion group on chronic fatigue syndrome for health professionals.

Subscribe CFS-MED Firstname Lastname

L **CFS-NEWS**

listserv@maelstrom.stjohns.edu

Electronic newsletter focusing on chronic fatigue syndrome.

Subscribe CFS-NEWS Firstname Lastname

W **Chronic Fatigue Syndrome (CFS)**

http://www.cais.com/cfs-news/

An impressive collection of links to CFS resources on the Net; compiled by Roger Burns, publisher of the CFS-NEWS Electronic Newsletter. FAQs, informational articles, discussion groups, and magazines are among the resources covered here.

Contact: Roger Burns, cfs-news@cais.cais.com

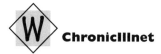 **ChronicIllnet**

http://www.chronicillnet.org/

ChronicIllnet is the first multimedia information source on the Internet dedicated to chronic illnesses including AIDS, cancer, Persian Gulf War syndrome, autoimmune diseases, chronic fatigue syndrome, heart disease, and neurological diseases. The information at this site is designed to appeal to a wide audience including researchers, physicians, and laypeople.

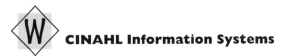

CINAHL Information Systems

http://cinahl.com/

The CINAHL Information Systems Website is a key access point to multidisciplinary professional literature. For nearly 40 years, nurses, health care professionals, researchers, students, and educators have known CINAHL as their number one resource for professional literature on the nursing, allied health, biomedical, and health care industries. CINAHL continues to expand its coverage and now includes nearly 800 journals and more than 215,000 records. You'll find detailed product profiles of all print, CD-ROM, online, and ancillary products in the CINAHL Products section. CINAHL direct online service is available, but does require the payment of a membership fee.

Contact: cinahl@cinahl.com

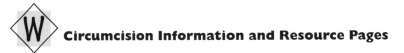

Circumcision Information and Resource Pages

http://www.cirp.org/CIRP/

The Circumcision Information and Resource Pages are an Internet resource, providing information about all aspects of the genital surgery known as circumcision. Whether or not circumcision should be performed is a controversial question, especially as religious issues may be involved. One of the aims of the Circumcision Information and Resource Pages is to provide parents with information to assist them, if and when they are confronted with this question.

Contact: Geoffrey T. Falk, gtf@cirp.org

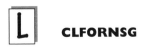

CLFORNSG

listserv@ulkyvm.louisville.edu

Discussion list for nurses interested in forensic nursing.

Subscribe CLFORNSG Firstname Lastname

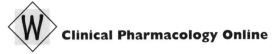

Clinical Pharmacology Online

http://www.cponline.gsm.com/

If you become a subscriber to this service, there is a wealth of drug information available. Nonsubscribers have less access, but they can still find answers to many drug-related questions. There is a searchable drug database that is very comprehensive.

Contact: http://www.cponline.gsm.com/

L CLINICAL-TRIAL-FINDER

listserv@garcia.com

Information on clinical trials nationwide.

Subscribe CTF Firstname Lastname

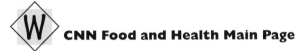

CNN Food and Health Main Page

http://www.cnn.com/HEALTH/

CNN has been a leader in news coverage around the world for 15 years. CNN online measures up to this standard by presenting features with full-text articles. The CNN Food and Health Main Page has full-text articles on the latest food and health news. Visitors cannot only read the articles but can also hear sound bites from salient interviews.

 ## CNSA-L

listserv@listserv.utoronto.ca

CNSA-L is a discussion group for CNSA/AEIC, the national bilingual voice of nursing students in diploma and baccalaureate programs in Canada.

Subscribe CNSA-L Firstname Lastname{/DIRCON}

L CNS-L

listserv@listserv.utoronto.ca

Discussion group for clinical nurse specialists, affiliated with the CNS Interest Group of Ontario, Canada.

Subscribe CNS-L Firstname Lastname

W College of Nursing and Health Science at George Mason University

http://www.ido.gmu.edu/departments/nursing/

Visitors to this site can find information on programs in the college, as well as *E-Dimensions,* the college publication; information on the Center for Outcomes Research and Data Analysis; and the Ethics Forum.

Contact: Veronica D. Feeg, rfeeg@gmu.edu

L COLON

listserv@listserv.acor.org

Discussion group on colon cancer and related issues.

Subscribe COLON Firstname Lastname

W Colorado Nurses' Association

http://www.sni.net/cna/

Home page of the Colorado Nurses' Association, with legislative news, member information, information on the state practice act, and listings of upcoming events.

Contact: Tim Brackett, RN, BSN, CNA@Nurses-CO.ORG

Columbia University Gastroenterology Web

http://cpmcnet.columbia.edu/dept/gi/

A good starting point to link to other sites with gastroenterology and liver disease information on the Internet.

Contact: Howard J.Worman, MD, hjw14@columbia.edu

Columbia University School of Nursing

http://cpmcnet.columbia.edu/dept/nursing/

Information on the School of Nursing at Columbia University in New York, with descriptions of programs, course listings, and faculty roster.

Contact: sonadmit@columbia.edu

Community Health Information Resources

http://chmis.org/

The Community Health Information Resources Website provides information for community-based health information partnerships such as CHIN (Community Health Information Networks), CHMIS (Community Health Management Information Systems), and RHIN (Regional Health Information Networks); employers, health plans, and health care providers interested in instituting quality measurement projects in their communities; and groups initiating health information studies, outcomes projects, and patient satisfaction studies. The Community Health Information Resources Website was developed under a grant from the John A. Hartford Foundation and is administered by the Foundation for Health Care Quality.

Contact: baguilar@eskimo.com

Community of Science Web Server

http://best.gdb.org/best.html

The Community of Science World Wide Web server contains information about scientific expertise, funded scientific research, and funding opportunities for research. The COS philosophy is to provide working researchers with valuable information tools to help them complete work underway and secure funds for the next project. COS is a consortium of research institutions and one of the largest repositories of searchable scientific information available on the Internet.

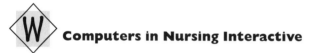

Computer Related Repetitive Strain Injury

http://engr-www.unl.edu/ee/eeshop/rsi.html

"Use a light touch when typing. Don't tightly squeeze the mouse. Take frequent breaks." These are among the tips for avoiding repetitive strain injury (RSI) found at this site, which also offers diagrams of proper typing position and descriptions of the first warning signs of injuries. The author of the page is Paul Marxhausen, an engineering electronics technician who has suffered from RSI since March 1994.

Contact: Paul Marxhausen, mpaul@unlinfo.unl.edu

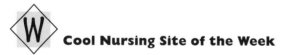

Computers in Nursing Interactive

http://www.cini.com

This site is dedicated to the interactive Web version of the journal *Computers in Nursing* and will feature up-to-date information and news about computer applications in nursing. Resources are provided here that are not available in the print version.

Contact: Leslie H. Nicoll, lnicoll@maine.maine.edu

Cool Nursing Site of the Week

http://www.odyssee.net/~fnord/nurselink.html

Although I have tried to be comprehensive in this guide, new sites appear daily. Visit the cool nursing site of the week to find out what is new, and cool, on the Web.

Contact: Thomas Moll, fnord@odyssee.net

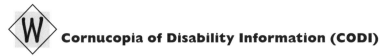

Cornucopia of Disability Information (CODI)

http://codi.buffalo.edu/

CODI serves as a community resource for consumers and professionals by providing disability information in a wide variety of areas. The information addresses university (State University of New York at Buffalo), local (Buffalo and western New York), state, national, and international audiences. Submissions are welcome from these communities. Areas include education, directories and databases, statistics, government documents, computer access, legal, publications, WWW, bibliographic references, aging, politics, universal design, and announcements.

Contact: Jay Leavitt, (leavitt@acsu.buffalo.edu)

Country Joe McDonald's Tribute to Florence Nightingale

http://www.dnai.com/~borneo/nightingale/

You have to see this site to believe it. The singer, Country Joe McDonald, has become a student of the life of Florence Nightingale. This site includes a history of Miss Nightingale, a picture of Country Joe's nurse doll collection, and the film treatment he is developing for a movie of Miss Nightingale's life. The entire site is beautifully done, with many pictures and a recording of Miss Nightingale, made in 1890 (the same recording that is available at InterNurse).

Contact: Country Joe McDonald, joe@www.countryjoe.com

L C-PALSY

listserv@maelstron.stjohns.edu

Discussion group about cerebral palsy and related issues.

Subscribe C-PALSY Firstname Lastname

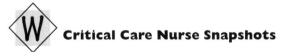

Critical Care Nurse Snapshots

http://www.nursing.ab.umd.edu/students/~jkohl/scenario/opening.htm

Critical Care Nurse Snapshots are designed to be interactive case scenarios for nurses involved in making informed decisions at the bedside. Each case study will involve the student in the critical thinking process as it relates to the assessment, diagnosis, management, and follow-up of a clinically based problem.

Contact: John Kohl, jkohl@umabnet.ab.umd.edu

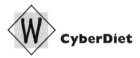 **CTNURS-L**

listserv@uconnvm.uconn.edu

Discussion list for the nurses of Connecticut.

Subscribe CTNURS-L Firstname Lastname

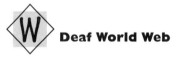 **CyberDiet**

http://www.cyberdiet.com

CyberDiet, "the best place to go to answer all your questions about adopting a healthy lifestyle," is the work of cofounders Timi Gustafson, RD, and Cynthia Fink. The site offers highly interactive modules that allow its users to customize a program to achieve their specific goals, as well as providing vast nutritional information at the click of a mouse. CyberDiet offers its visitors a means of achieving their specific goals through extensive use of online interactive modules as well as detailed nutritional information and motivation.

Contact: eatright@cyberdiet.com

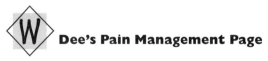 **Deaf World Web**

http://dww.deafworldweb.org/

Deaf and hearing people alike can click into the world of the deaf at this expanding site. The site includes news, an encyclopedia, dicussion and chat areas, information for children, and an interactive American Sign Language (ASL) dictionary.

Contact: dww@deafworldweb.org

W **Dee's Pain Management Page**

http://www.web-shack.com/dee/

Dee Burrows is a nurse, teacher, and researcher at Buckinghamshire College of Nursing and Midwifery. Her home page includes her own experience with and research on pain management, information on the Pain Interest Group of South Buckinghamshire, and other nursing and pain management links.

Contact: Dee Burrows, dee@ptop.demon.co.uk

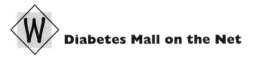 **DEA — Department of Justice**

http://www.usdoj.gov/dea/index.htm

Home page for the Drug Enforcement Agency (DEA) of the Department of Justice. Includes information on the mission of the DEA, programs, education, and fugitives. Information regarding distribution of controlled substances for medicinal purposes can be found under "Diversion" in the programs section.

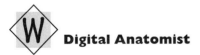 **Diabetes Mall on the Net**

http://www.diabetesnet.com/

Founded in 1993 by John Walsh, PA CDE, and Ruth Roberts, MA, Diabetes Services develops products and services, such as educational materials, software, and news updates for people who have diabetes. A complete list of persons affiliated with Diabetes Services can be found at http://www.diabetesnet.com/dauthors.html.

Contact: contact@diabetesnet.com

différance: Peter Murray's Home Page

http://www.lemmus.demon.co.uk/diff01.htm

This Website has links to nursing informatics topics related to nursing and health care informatics, journals, people, and sites. Also includes links to the Betty Neuman page with information about the theorist and the Neuman Systems Model.

Contact: p.j.murray@open.ac.uk

Digital Anatomist

http://www1.biostr.washington.edu/DigitalAnatomist.html

A virtual anatomy lab with hundreds of images.

Contact: digital_anatomist@biostr.washington.edu

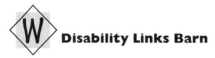 **Disability Links Barn**

http://www.accessunlimited.com/links.html

A site of links for people with disabilities of all types. The site is well organized and comprehensive. It is sponsored by Access Unlimited, a manufacturer and distributor of adaptive transportation and mobility equipment for people with disabilities.

Contact: accessun@spectra.net

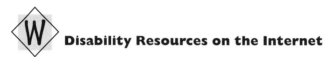 **Disability Resources on the Internet**

http://disability.com/

Disability Resources on the Internet is an index compiled by Evan Kemp Associates, a company based in Washington, DC. The index is well organized with categories such as Disability Related Legal Resources and Health and Medicine Resources.

Contact: webmaster@disability.com

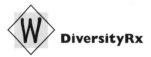 **Diseases, Disorders and Related Topics**

http://www.mic.ki.se/Diseases/index.html

An exhaustive collection of resources for laypeople, health care professionals, and scientists involved in the study or treatment of diseases, disorders, or any number of related medical issues. Whether your specialty is bacterial, behavioral, viral, or parasitic, in the realm of animal diseases, anesthesia, surgery, or dentistry, the Karolinska Institute's Diseases, Disorders and Related Topics is sure to cover it. Of special interest is a humanities section exploring ethics in medicine.

Contact: tor.ahlenius@mic.ki.se

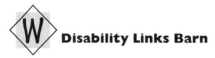 **DiversityRx**

http://www.diversityrx.org/HTML/DIVRX.htm

DiversityRx promotes language and cultural competence to improve the quality of health care for minority, immigrant, and ethnically diverse communities. This site has many resources in support of that mission.

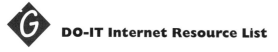

DO-IT Internet Resource List

gopher://hawking.u.washington.edu

The DO-IT Gopher is maintained by Project DO-IT (Disabilities, Opportunities, Internetworking, and Technology) at the University of Washington. The DO-IT program is primarily funded by the National Science Foundation. Its purpose is to increase participation of individuals with disabilities in academic programs and careers in science, engineering, and mathematics. The DO-IT Gopher is designed for people who are interested in this effort. Students with disabilities; parents; precollege teachers and counselors; service providers; employers; and postsecondary staff and faculty in science, engineering, and mathematics are welcome. The Gopher includes resources related to disability, science, engineering, mathematics, postsecondary education, and careers.

Contact: doit@u.washington.edu

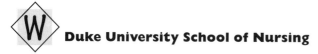

Duke University School of Nursing

http://son3.mc.duke.edu/

This Website has program, faculty, educational resources, and contact information at the Duke University School of Nursing.

Contact: webmaster@son3.mc.duke.edu

East Tennessee State University College of Nursing

http://www.east-tenn-st.edu/etsucon/

This Website has program information, news, and nursing-related links.

Contact: etsucon@nursserv.east-tenn-st.edu

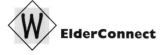

ElderConnect

http://www.extendedcare.com/

The ElderConnect database contains information about more than 33,000 acute rehabilitation providers, retirement communities, and providers specializing in all levels of long-term nursing care as well as home health agencies. This database can help you research such providers and agencies by performing a search using criteria such as geographic location and type of care required. You will quickly find the provider of extended care that you are seeking.

Contact: ecininc@ecininc.com{/DIRCON}

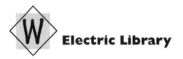 **Electric Library**

http://www.elibrary.com/id/2525/

The Electric Library is a searchable database. With the Electric Library, any person can pose a question in plain English and launch a comprehensive, simultaneous search through more than 150 full-text newspapers, hundreds and hundreds of full-text magazines, two international newswires, two thousand classic books, hundreds of maps, thousands of photographs, as well as major works of literature and art. To use this search engine, you must subscribe to the service, and there is a fee, although trial subscriptions are available.

Contact: elibrary@infonautics.com

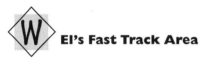 **EI's Fast Track Area**

http://www.geocities.com/HotSprings/1003/

Eleanor Elston is a registered nurse working in an emergency department of a large teaching hospital in British Columbia. Her home page includes a variety of nursing links, personal information, and some humorous sites.

Contact: eelston@iname.com

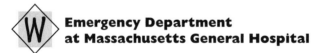 **Emergency Department at Massachusetts General Hospital**

http://emergency.mgh.harvard.edu/

Test your diagnostic skills against practitioners from around the world. The Interesting Case Conference presents a series of cases. Figure out the diagnosis and e-mail in your answer, or join the Emergency Bulletin Board to discuss the case.

Contact: Pierre Borczuk, MD, %20pierreb@highway1.com

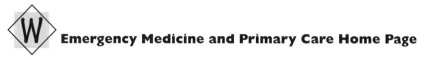
Emergency Medicine and Primary Care Home Page

http://www.embbs.com/

Educational resources for emergency and primary care providers. The site includes radiologic images, CT scans, and a megacode simulator.

Contact: Ash Nashed, MD, ashrafn@aol.com

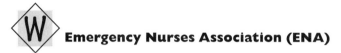
Emergency Nurses Association (ENA)

http://www.ena.org/

The ENA home page highlights information about the association, the ENA foundation, the Board of Certification for Emergency Nursing, and EN C.A.R.E. (Cancel Alcohol Related Emergencies).

Contact: ENAinfo@ena.org

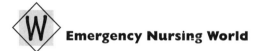
Emergency Nursing World

http://www.wenet.net/~ttrimble/enw/enw_toc.html

Lots of information for nurses in emergency practice. The tips and tricks are particularly useful.

Contact: Tom Trimble, RN, ttrimble@hooked.net

EM-NSG-L

listserv@itssrv1.itsa.ucsf.edu

Discussion list for emergency nurses.

Subscribe EM-NSG-L Firstname Lastname

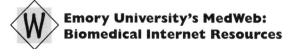
Emory University's MedWeb: Biomedical Internet Resources

http://www.cc.emory.edu/WHSCL/medweb.html

Emory University's MedWeb is a list of more than 8,000 links to health information Web pages. The table of contents includes pages on AIDS, cardiology, educational resources, grants and funding, nursing, and public health. The nursing page has links to schools of nursing and career directories, Websites, documents, and electronic newsletters and journals.

Contact: Steve Foote, libsf@emory.edu

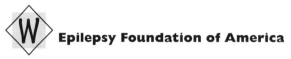

Epilepsy Foundation of America

http://www.efa.org/indexf.htm

Home page for the Epilepsy Foundation of America. The site includes information for patients, family members, and health professionals in the areas of research, advocacy, education, and service. There is information on the Gene Discovery Project and a special "Kid's Korner."

Contact: wilsona@efa.org

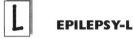

EPILEPSY-L

listserv@home.ease.lsoft.com

Discussion group about epilepsy and seizure disorders.

Subscribe EPILEPSY-L Firstname Lastname

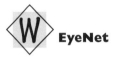

EyeNet

http://www.eyenet.org/

An education and reference site maintained by the American Academy of Ophthalmology, an international member association of more than 21,000 specialists. A visit to EyeNet will help you resolve the eternal question, "What's the difference between an Optometrist and an Optician?" as well as questions you may have about eye conditions such as macular degeneration and glaucoma. The academy also maintains a Member Services area that provides news for AAO members.

Contact: webmaster@aao.org

EYENURSE

Discussion group for nurses practicing in ophthalmology.

Contact Linda Vader, lavader@umich.edu for subscription information.

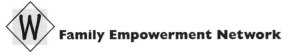

Family Empowerment Network

http://www.downsyndrome.com/

Maintained by Cindy and Timothy Casten (their son, Mattie, has Down syndrome, DS), this site offers families and friends of individuals with DS valuable information about the genetic disorder while advocating for the rights of the disabled. The site offers a wealth of information relating to the disorder's genetic basis, health concerns, research news, updates of government programs and legislative news, educational resources, information about support networks (both on- and off-line), and personal accounts from parents and siblings of individuals with DS. It is also a valuable site for parents of a newborn child with Down syndrome.

Contact: Cindy and Timothy Casten, TCasten@downsyndrome.com

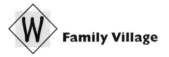

Family Village

http://www.familyvillage.wisc.edu/tindex.htm

The Family Village is a global community that integrates information, resources, and communication opportunities on the Internet for persons with cognitive and other disabilities, their families, and those who provide them services and supports. The Family Village Website has a well-rounded offering of information for disabled persons including medical, educational, spiritual, and recreational resources.

Contact: rowley@waisman.wisc.edu

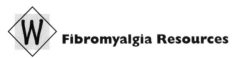

Fedworld

telnet://fedworld.gov/

A U.S. government–maintained database of documents and resources on a wide variety of topics including health, medicine, and nursing.

Fibromyalgia Resources

http://www.hsc.missouri.edu/fibro/fibrotp.html

The Missouri Arthritis Rehabilitation Research and Training Center has created this Website as an educational resource for patients and physicians. This site has fibromyalgia FAQs for patients and health care providers, other education resources, and information about their organization.

Contact: Susan Hazelwood, susan_hazelwood@mailsvr.hsc.missouri.edu

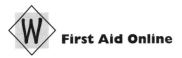 **First Aid Online**

http://www.prairienet.org/~autumn/firstaid/

Ever wonder how prepared you would be in a home emergency situation? First Aid Online prepares readers with instructions on the appropriate reactions to and actions in any of a list of common crises. Choking, burns, poisoning, and frostbite are only a few of the ailments covered in this very handy, easy-to-read guide to safety.

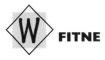 **FITNE**

http://www.ev.net/fitne/

FITNE promotes the use of technology in health care education by developing and distributing multimedia hardware systems and software. The home page has information on the conferences, products, seminars, and more.

Contact: webmaster@fitne.ev.net

Florida Atlantic University College of Nursing

http://www.fau.edu/divdept/nursing/nur.htm

This site includes a description of programs, faculty listing with research interests, and back issues of "Nightingale Songs," a publication that allows nurses to "share their silent moments of reflection on their nursing."

Contact: Lenora Pitts, lpitts@acc.fau.edu

Florida International University School of Nursing

http://www.fiu.edu/orgs/nursing/

Informational site with course descriptions, faculty listing, and programs. The site also includes information on a number of nursing theories and a bibliography of readings on Orem.

Contact: Douglas Coffin, PhD, ARNP, coffin@fiu.edu

W Florida State University School of Nursing

http://www.fsu.edu/~nursing/Nursing.html

This site has information on the degree programs, course requirements, faculty, and a description and history of the school of nursing.

Contact: WebMaster, scoughli@mailer.fsu.edu

W Fort Hays State University School of Nursing

http://www.fhsu.edu/nursing/

This site includes information on courses, programs, and faculty. In addition, there is an online continuing education course on Acute Otitis Media. Plans call for more courses to be added in the future.

Contact: Pam Sexton, nups@bigcat.fhsu.edu

W Frances Payne Bolton School of Nursing

http://fpb.cwru.edu

Visitors here can learn about the Frances Payne Bolton School of Nursing at Case Western Reserve University. The site includes information from the general bulletin, faculty listing, degree programs, and curriculum information. It is also possible to browse a list of course-related resources (notes, syllabi, news groups, and so on) for the school of nursing and learn more about NurseWeb, started by students at FPB.

Contact: aurora@po.cwru.edu

W Galaxy

http://www.einet.net/galaxy.html

Galaxy is a guide to worldwide services and information, sponsored by Trade-Wave Corporation. The site provides links to many topics of interest, including business, community, engineering, government, humanities, law, leisure, medicine, reference, science, and the social sciences. Although many of the links from the nursing section have been explored and included elsewhere in this directory, this is a good site to connect to many other areas of information.

Contact: galaxy@tradewave.com

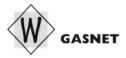 **GASNET**

http://gasnet.med.yale.edu

GASNET is a global anesthesiology server network that includes a multimedia textbook, *Educational Synopses in Anesthesiology and Critical Care Medicine;* the first electronic journal of anesthesiology; abstracts from several journals; commercial software demonstrations; an e-mail directory; and links to many other anesthesiology resources on the Internet.

Contact: Keith J. Ruskin, webmaster@gasnet.med.yale.edu

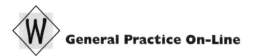 **General Practice On-Line**

http://www.cityscape.co.uk/users/ad88/gp.htm

The site of the *International Journal of General Practice and Primary Care,* a peer-reviewed electronic journal with articles for primary care providers. There are also links to other electronic journals published by Priory Lodge Education, including *Chest Medicine On-Line, Dentistry On-Line, Psychiatry On-Line,* and *Family Medicine On-Line.*

 GERINET

listserv@listserv.acsu.buffalo.edu

Discussion group for geriatric care, gerontology, and related issues.

Subscribe GERINET Firstname Lastname

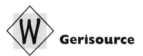 **Gerisource**

http://www.gerisource.com/

Gerisource is a multidiscipinary clinical bulletin designed for those who work in long-term care. This site includes articles and information on geriatrics, aging, and long-term care.

Contact: info@gerisource.com

GERO-NURSE

GERO-NURSE-REQUEST@list.uiowa.edu

Listserv for the Research Development and Dissemination Core at the University of Iowa Gerontological Nursing Intervention Research Center.

Subscribe

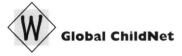 **Global ChildNet**

http://edie.cprost.sfu.ca/gcnet/index.html

Global ChildNet, with its headquarters in Vancouver, BC, was officially introduced at the Child Health 2000 World Congress. It is an organization that uses the Internet to offer a range of easily accessible, child health–related online services. These services include databases and other information on issues related to the well-being of the world's children. As a division of the Global Child Health Society, a nonprofit organization, Global ChildNet also publishes an on-line version of the *Global Child Health News and Review,* as well as supplying information on the Child Health 2000 World Congress and Exposition. By using state-of-the-art technology, Global ChildNet complements the newspaper and the congress to provide worldwide networking for health professionals, child health workers, scientists, nongovernmental organizations, health planners, and child advocates.

Contact: gcnet@unixg.ubc.ca

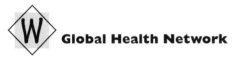 **Global Health Network**

http://www.pitt.edu/HOME/GHNet/GHNet.html#r4

The mission of the GHN is to develop a world wide network of people engaged in public health and disease prevention. Information at the site is available in Japanese, Spanish, Portugese, German, Chinese and Turkish, as well as English.

Contact: Amy Brenen brenena@ghnet.org

 GLOBALRN

LISTSERV@ITSSRV1.UCSF.EDU

Discussion of topics related to culture and health for all interested health care professionals. Note: at one time this list was named CULTURE-AND-HEALTH;

you may still see references to that list on the Internet, but this list, GLOBALRN, is the one you should subscribe to.

Subscribe GLOBALRN Firstname Lastname

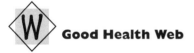 **GlobalRN Website**

http://nurseweb.ucsf.edu/www/globalrn.htm

GLOBALRN is a worldwide Internet e-mail discussion list on culture and health care issues. This page is maintained by the list owner (supervisor) of GLOBALRN to highlight World Wide Web resources of interest in these subject areas.

Contact: Chuck Pitkofsy, chuckp@itsa.ucsf.edu

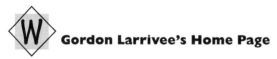 **Good Health Web**

http://www.social.com/health/index.html

The Good Health Web contains various health resources including an annotated database of more than 1,000 health organizations, health information, FAQs, and links to other sites. A visitor here will learn to access information on the Internet using different forums, such as interactive discussions (posts and read only), links, and mailing lists.

Contact: webmaster@social.com

Gordon Larrivee's Home Page

http://www.ummed.edu/pub/l/larrivee/home.html

Gordon Larrivee is a specialist in nursing informatics at the University of Massachusetts Medical Center. He currently holds an associate faculty appointment at the U Mass Graduate School of Nursing. He is an active member of Boston Area Nursing Informatics Consortium (BANIC) and is the owner and editor of Nrsing-L, a mailing list for the discussion of nursing informatics.

Contact: Gordon Larrivee, gordon.larrivee@ummed.edu

Greyhound-L

LISTSERV@MAIL.EWORLD.COM

Exclusively dedicated to Greyhounds, both retired racers and others.

Subscribe Greyhound-L Firstname Lastname

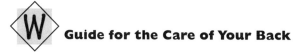 ## Guide for the Care of Your Back

http://www.halcyon.com/moonbeam/back/

An illustrated guide to proper care of one's back, courtesy of the Virginia Mason Medical Center. With remarkable thoroughness, the guide demonstrates strategies for sitting, standing, bending, lying down, and lifting that place the least stress on the vertebrae, ligaments, and muscles that compose the back. If you're too busy to visit the site, remember this: "Slouching is unacceptable."

Contact: William Julien, moonbeam@catmanor.com

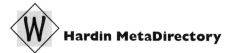 ## Hardin MetaDirectory

http://www.lib.uiowa.edu/hardin-www/md-idx.html

"We list the sites that list the sites." The original and perhaps the most complete index on the Web. Brought to you courtesy of the Hardin Library for the Health Sciences at the University of Iowa.

Contact: Eric Rumsey, eric-rumsey@uiowa.edu

 ## HCARENURS

listserv@listserv.medec.com

Discussion group for home care nurses.

Subscribe HCARENURS Firstname Lastname

HCFA: The Medicare and Medicaid Agency

http://www.hcfa.gov/

Visitors to the Medicare and Medicaid site will find such resources as *Healthcare Financing News,* the Medicare Q&A for 85 common questions, and a survey of research and demonstration initiatives.

Contact: webmaster@hcfa.gov

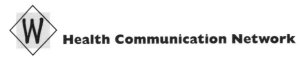

Healthcare Information Systems Directory

http://www.health-infosys-dir.com/

The Healthcare Information Systems Directory provides one-stop shopping for hospitals, clinics, HMOs, PPOs, and other health care providers. Browse through an updated list of vendors who supply particular types of software and compare their strengths with your needs.

Contact: hisd@health-infosys-dir.com

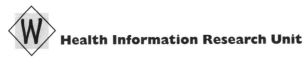

Health Communication Network

http://www.hcn.net.au/

From Australia, a site providing a variety of health and biomedical information.

Contact: hcn@hcn.net.au

Health Information Research Unit

http://hiru.mcmaster.ca/

Investigators, staff, and associates of the Health Information Research Unit (HIRU), Department of Clinical Epidemiology and Biostatistics, Faculty of Health Sciences, McMaster University, study the phenomenology of health information, develop information tools to support evidence-based care, and evaluate informational health interventions. They share this information with the world community of health professionals through this Website.

Contact: haywardr@fhs.mcmaster.ca

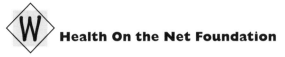 **Health On the Net Foundation**

http://www.hon.ch/HomePage/Home-Page.html

An international initiative, Health On the Net Foundation is a nonprofit organization, headquartered in Geneva, Switzerland. The foundation is dedicated to realizing the benefits of the Internet and related technologies in the fields of medicine and health care. With private and public sector support, the foundation actively promotes effective Internet use and demonstrates best-in-class implementation and application. Visitors to this site can find information on the HON Initiative and the HON Code principles.

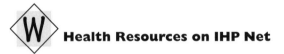 **Health Organizations**

http://www.social.com/health/nhic/data/index.html

This site provides a U.S. goverment database of more than 1,000 health organizations, including mailing address and, when available, e-mail contact information. The database can be searched by keyword, browsed alphabetically, or browsed by state.

 Health Resources on IHP Net

http://www.interaccess.com/ihpnet/health.html

Health Resources is a gateway to information on specific diseases, child health, substance abuse, health agencies, and other health resources on the Internet. Because it is inclusive of many different types of health information, this page is a good place to start a search.

Contact: ulysses@interaccess.com

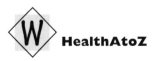 **HealthAtoZ**

http://www.healthAtoZ.com/

This site includes links and news. It is a search site, designed specifically for health professionals.

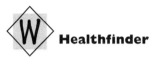 **Healthcare Informatics Standards**

http://www.mcis.duke.edu/standards/guide.htm

This site is a catalog of information about health care informatics standards. The site provides valuable information to those who regularly work in this area, but it also features introductory material for health care professionals who are new to informatics or standards.

Contact: Al Stone, stone001@mc.duke.edu

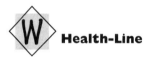 **Healthfinder**

http://www.healthfinder.gov

Healthfinder is a gateway consumer health and human services information Website from the United States government. Healthfinder can lead you to se-lected online publications, clearinghouses, databases, Websites, and support and self-help groups, as well as the government agencies and not-for-profit organizations that produce reliable information for the public.

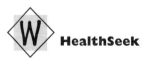 **Health-Line**

http://www.health-line.org/index2.html

Informative site on health insurance, brought to you by the Life and Health Insurance Foundation for Education. The glossary of 25 health insurance terms is particularly helpful.

Contact: info@life-line.org

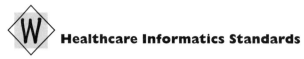 **HealthSeek**

http://www.healthseek.com/

HealthSeek is a commercial online health care information service, providing health care professionals, consumers, and companies with a central site for ob-taining news, information, and resources.

Contact: fisher@healthseek.com

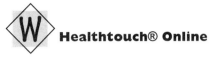 **Healthtouch® Online**

http://www.healthtouch.com

Healthtouch® Online brings together information from various health organizations. Visitors to this page may conduct searches to find drug information or listings (not necessarily complete) of local pharmacies. The Health Resource Directory lists the health organizations and health government agencies that provide information on Healthtouch® Online. Health information is available on topics that include the prevention and treatment of AIDS, asthma, diet and nutrition, drug and alcohol abuse, eye diseases, mental health, and poison prevention.

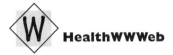 **HealthWWWeb**

http://www.healthwwweb.com/healthwwweb.html

HealthWWWeb is a site that combines integrative medicine, natural health, and alternative therapies. The site includes information on nutrition and healing therapies and links to other health-oriented sites on the WWW. Links to AMR'TA, the Alchemical Medicine Research and Teaching Association, are also included at this site.

Contact:Webmaster@HealthWWWeb.com

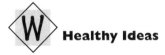 **Healthy Ideas**

http://www.healthyideas.com/index.html

Healthy Ideas is brought to you by *Prevention Magazine,* the popular health magazine published by Rodale. The site is organized into four main channels: Natural Living offers information on natural health treatments, including herbs, vitamins, and news; Weight Loss & Fitness emphasizes healthy, empowering weight management techniques; Healthy Cooking includes recipes and nutrition news. Click on Healthy Cooking; and Family Health includes parenting advice and clinical information.

HEM-ONC

listserv@listserv.acor.org

Discussion group for hematologic oncology. Professionally oriented.

Subscribe HEM-ONC Firstname Lastname

 **HepNet**

http://www.hepnet.com/index.html

This site focuses on the needs of the medical community, providing updates on patient care issues, serology, new clinical papers, and news releases, as well as links to many other excellent hepatitis-related sites.

Contact: Webmaster@hepnet.com

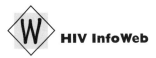 **HIV InfoWeb**

http://www.infoweb.org/

Links, articles, and other resources on HIV and AIDS.

 HODGKINS

listserv@solar.org

Discussion group on Hodgkin's disease and related lymphomas.

Subscribe HODGKINS (do not follow by typing your name)

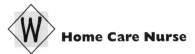 **Home Care Nurse**

http://junior.apk.net/~nurse/

This page grew out of the hcarenurs (Home Care Nurse) Listserv, which provides a platform for home care nurses to discuss clinical, ethical, and administrative issues. This page contains links to other Web pages and Listservs of interest to home care nurses.

Contact: Liz Madigan, eam13@po.cwru.edu

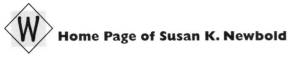

Home Page of Susan K. Newbold

http://www.nursing.ab.umd.edu//students/~snewbol/

Susan K. Newbold's Website has information on CARING (Capital Area Round-table on Informatics in NursinG), links to Computers in Nursing–Interactive, Nursing Informatics and Health Informatics Conferences, nursing informatics FAQs, and lists of nursing informatics groups around the world and nursing organizations and publications with e-mail access. A visitor here can also link to organizational information on the Pi Chapter of Sigma Theta Tau International Nursing Honor Society.

Contact: Susan Newbold, snewbold@umabnet.ab.umd.edu

HOMECAREQUAL

listserv@listserv.medec.com

Discussion group on home care quality.

Subscribe HOMECAREQUAL Firstname Lastname

HOMEHLTH

listserv@list.iex.net

Discussion group on home health care and related issues.

Subscribe HOMEHLTH Firstname Lastname

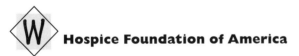

Hospice Foundation of America

http://www.hospicefoundation.org/

On this page you can learn about hospice care, how to select a hospice, and how to locate a hospice near you. You can learn of the Hospice Foundation's programs, read excerpts from their publications, order books and videos, and sign up for the annual bereavement teleconference.

Contact: hospicefdn@charitiesusa.org

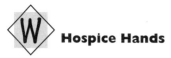 **Hospice Hands**

http://hospice-cares.com/

An online hospice community, sponsored by Hospice of North Central Florida. Lots of resources about hospice and links to other hospice sites.

Contact: healing@hospice-cares.com

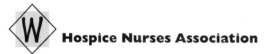 **Hospice Nurses Association**

http://www.Roxane.COM/HNA

Home page of the Hospice Nurses Association.

Contact: hnafan@pipeline.com

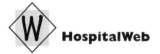 **HospitalWeb**

http://neuro-www.mgh.harvard.edu/hospitalweb.nclk

HospitalWeb is a growing list of hospitals on the Web. Providing a simple and globally accessible way for patients, medical researchers, and physicians to get information on any hospital in the world is the goal. This list is of "main" Web servers (only Web servers at hospitals) as opposed to departments within hospitals. The site is maintained by the Department of Neurology at Massachusetts General Hospital.

Contact: lester@helix.mgh.harvard.edu

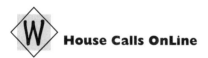 **House Calls OnLine**

http://iswest.net/~quan/housecalls.html

A telezine for home health care professionals, with articles, patient and safety tips, and hot links.

Contact: Kathy Quan, RN, BSN, PHN, housecalls-online@juno.com

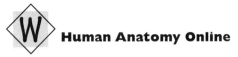 Human Anatomy Online

http://www.InnerBody.com/

A colorful, interactive human anatomy site. You can explore body systems that include full descriptions and other related illustrations.

 I-CAN

maiser@hoffman.mgen.pitt.edu

Listserv and discussion group of the Children's Amputee Network.

Subscribe I-CAN

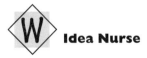 Idaho State University Department of Nursing

http://www.isu.edu/departments/nursing/

Highlights of this home page include information on the nursing program, faculty, student nurses association, and a newsnet. There are also links to other nursing newsgroups, Listservs, and Websites.

Contact: hewebeve@ucs.isu.edu

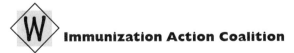 Idea Nurse

http://ideanurse.com/

Peter Ramme is an "idea nurse" who has successfully combined nursing experience with his knowledge of computers in providing continuing education. His page contains current events and pointers to nursing resources.

Contact: Peter Ramme, peter@silcom.com

Immunization Action Coalition

http://www.immunize.org/index.htm

Immunization Action Coalition, a 501(c)3 nonprofit organization, works to boost immunization rates in the United States. The coalition promotes physician, community, and family awareness of and responsibility for appropriate immunization of all people of all ages against all vaccine-preventable diseases. The coalition's WWW home page provides people with electronic versions of its newsletters, Needle Tips and Hepatitis B Coalition News, as well a mailing address to its organization on the Internet.

Contact: editor@immunize.org

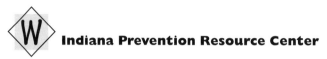

Indiana Prevention Resource Center

http://www.drugs.indiana.edu/druginfo/home.html

The center offers information about alcohol, tobacco, and drug abuse including a dictionary of slang terms, abbreviations, and acronyms compiled by the Indiana Prevention Resource Center and the National Drugs and Crime Clearinghouse files. Major headings include arguments against drug legalization, information on drug testing, workplace issues, and the Addiction Research Foundation's "Facts About" series and bibliographies.

Contact: webmaster@www.drugs.indiana.edu

Indiana University School of Nursing–Bloomington

http://www.indiana.edu/~iubnurse/nurse.html

The Indiana University School of Nursing home page has information on its academic programs, faculty, the Association of Nursing Students, and a bulletin board for students. There are also links to nursing-related Websites and sites of general interest.

Indiana University School of Nursing (Indianapolis)

http://www.iupui.edu/~nursing/index.html

Indiana University School of Nursing (IUSON) is an academic community internationally known for the excellence and diversity of its programs. One of the top-ranked and largest schools of nursing in the United States, IUSON awards the full range of academic degrees, from the associate to doctoral level, and offers courses on eight campuses throughout the state of Indiana. In addition, IUSON is actively developing a distance learning program using a variety of methodologies, including the Internet. Their Website has information about this initiative.

Contact: Louise Bowman, lbowman@wpo.iupui.edu

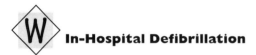

INDIE: The Integrated Network of Disability Information and Education

http://indie.ca

INDIE facilitates the sharing of disability-related information to foster a collaborative approach to addressing disability issues among Canadians with disabilities and their organizations.

Contact: webmaster@indie.ca

In-Hospital Defibrillation

http://www.defib.net

Should nurses do defibrillation? Read some views and issues at this site to make up your mind.

Contact: John Stewart, RN, MA, rn@defib.net

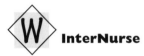

InterNurse

http://www.kencomp.net/internurse/

This site is designed to bring a sense of a nursing magazine to the Internet. There are many wonderful nurse-related sites and groups on the Net; Inter Nurse provides coverage for many of them. The site also gives the visitor useful nursing links in a separate section. One of the best things at this site is a recording of Florence Nightingale from 1890. You can actually listen to her voice!

Contact: Paul Mangan, internurse@dialin.net

International Association for the Study of Pain (IASP)

http://weber.u.washington.edu/%7Ecrc/IASP.html

The purposes of this Website are to introduce health care professionals and scientists to IASP, to provide services and resources to IASP members, to provide a vehicle for the educational outreach of IASP, to call attention to the importance of pain as a field for multidisciplinary scientific inquiry, and to make pain prevention and relief a priority for health care delivery.

Contact: C. Richard Chapman, PhD, crc@u.washington.edu

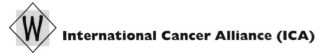

International Cancer Alliance (ICA)

http://www2.ari.net/icare/

The International Cancer Alliance (ICA) is a nonprofit organization that assists physicians, cancer patients and their families, and support groups in assuring that new, high-quality, focused, patient-centered cancer information is available to support the needs of each patient and physician. ICA has developed these programs through its education organization, the International Cancer Academy for Research and Education (ICARE). This organization is operated by a network of people: world-class scientists; clinicians; caring staff; and lay volunteers, many of whom are patients themselves. This Website has links to cancer patient information, ICARE programs, background on ICA, and a sign-up area for ICARE programs.

Contact: sysent@ari.net

International Committee of the Red Cross

http://www.icrc.ch/

A look at the work of the International Committee of the Red Cross, based in Geneva, Switzerland. The ICRC server features extensive information on Red Cross operations worldwide; the mission, philosophy, and strategic operations of the ICRC; issues and topics of concern to the organization; and a full explanation of International Humanitarian Law, including the full texts of the Geneva Conventions.

Contact: webmaster.gva@gwn.icrc.org

International Federation of MS Societies (IFMSS)

http://www.ifmss.org.uk/index.htm

IFMSS is a nongovernmental, nonprofit voluntary health agency and umbrella organization for the 34 established national MS member societies throughout the world. One of the major IFMSS objectives is to serve as a clearinghouse for educational and scientific information about MS. The World of Multiple Sclerosis (WoMS) is an international cooperative effort using experts in all areas of MS to offer current and useful information to all members of the MS community (health professionals, researchers, persons with MS, families, and caregivers), as well as the general public. The annotated directory has links to news and updates, research, user and support groups, publications, and other useful information.

Contact: Webmaster, psherida@extro.ucc.su.oz.au

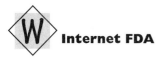 **International Food Information Council**

http://ificinfo.health.org/

The purpose of the International Food Information Council (IFIC) Foundation is to provide sound, scientific information on food safety and nutrition to journalists, health professionals, educators, government officials, and consumers. IFIC is a nonprofit organization based in Washington, DC. Information available includes scientific research, informational materials, graphics, and other information on a broad range of food issues. Some highlights include tips for teachers and consumers, a section containing information for reporters, answers to frequently asked food-related questions, and results from recent Gallup surveys.

Contact: foodinfo@ific.health.org

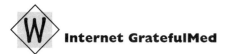 **Internet FDA**

http://www.fda.gov/fdahomepage.html

Assessing risks—and, for drugs and medical devices, weighing risks against benefits—is at the core of FDA's public health protection duties. By ensuring that products and producers meet certain standards, FDA protects consumers and enables them to know what they're buying. For example, the agency requires that drugs, both prescription and over-the-counter, be proven safe and effective.

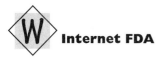 **Internet GratefulMed**

http://igm.nlm.nih.gov

Internet GratefulMed offers assisted searching in MEDLINE and other online databases of the U.S. National Library of Medicine (NLM). It was developed through the User Access Services project of NLM's System Reinvention initiative. Internet GratefulMed can map user terms through NLM's Unified Medical Language System® (UMLSR®). The Metathesaurus® helps users create, submit, and refine a search in MEDLINE. There is no charge to search MEDLINE using Internet GratefulMed. This new policy was implemented in June 1997.

Contact: Internet GratefulMed Development Team, access@nlm.nih.gov

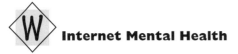

Internet Mental Health

http://www.mentalhealth.com

Internet Mental Health is a free encyclopedia of mental health information. It was developed by a Canadian psychiatrist, Phillip W. Long, and programmed by his colleague, Brian Chow. Their hope is that Internet Mental Health will promote improved understanding, diagnosis, and treatment of mental illness throughout the world.

Contact: editor@mentalhealth.com

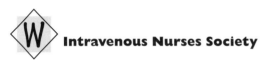

Intravenous Nurses Society

http://www.ins1.org/

The Intravenous Nurses Society exists to promote excellence in intravenous nursing through standards, education, public awareness, and research. INS's ultimate goal is to ensure access to the highest quality, cost-effective care for all individuals requiring and patients receiving intravenous therapies in all practice settings worldwide. This site is a resource of information on INS.

iNurse

http://www.inurse.com/

A specialty nursing site, created by Anthony J. Jannetti, Inc., publisher of *Nursing Economic$, MEDSURG Nursing,* and other professional journals.

Contact: Todd C. Lockhart, lockhart@voicenet.com

ITD-JNL

listserv@maelstrom.stjohns.edu

Electronic distribution of the *Information and Technology for the Disabled Journal.*

Subscribe ITD-JNL Firstname Lastname

ITNA

listserv@listserv.bcm.tmc.edu

Discussion list for the International TeleNurses Association.

Subscribe ITNA Firstname Lastname

 IVTHERAPY-L

listserv@netcom.com

Discussion list for IV therapy nurse clinicians.

Subscribe ivtherapy-1@netcom.com Firstname Lastname

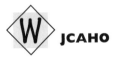 **Jack's Sunshine Nurse's Site**

http://www.mauigateway.com/~jackw/

Jack Wells' home page, described as a site developed for nurses by nurses. Dedicated to addressing issues that are relevent to nurses and the public concerning health care.

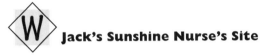 **JCAHO**

http://www.jcaho.org/

This Website, from the Joint Commission on Accreditation of Healthcare Organizations, is designed to inform the health care community and the public about the Joint Commission, its services, and its products. Information is updated regularly to reflect the ongoing changes in health. The Quality Calendar has a new quality quote every day.

Contact: webmaster@jcaho.org

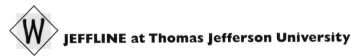 **JEFFLINE at Thomas Jefferson University**

http://Jeffline.tju.edu/

JEFFLINE is the entry point to Thomas Jefferson University WWW information service. The clever interface—it looks like an office—directs you to points of interest. For example, the books on the shelf take you to the library, the calendar on the bulletin board takes you to current events, and the lab coat on the hook in the corner takes you to patient care resources.

Contact: apollo@jeflin.tju.edu

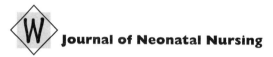
Johns Hopkins University School of Nursing

http://sonnet.nsg.jhu.edu/

Information on the school of nursing, the faculty, courses, and programs. Within the Center for Nursing Research is a useful document with tips on writing a successful grant application. Also, the school of nursing recently moved into a new building. Pictures of their new home are online.

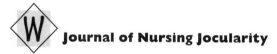
Journal of Neonatal Nursing

http://www.bizjet.com/jnn/

The electronic version of the *Journal of Neonatal Nursing* is the official journal of the UK Neonatal Nurses Association and the journal for all professionals who care for neonates and their families. Included are abstracts of all the articles published in the current issue of the journal, as well as one complete article from each issue.

Contact: jnn@bizjet.com

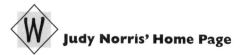
Journal of Nursing Jocularity

http://www.jocularity.com/toc.html

The online version of this journal features articles and cartoons that focus on the humorous aspects of the nursing profession. A stop here will tickle your funny bone.

Contact: 104645.2764@compuserve.com

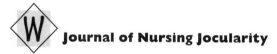
Judy Norris' Home Page

http://www.ualberta.ca/~jrnorris/

Judy Norris' Website contains the QualPage, resources related to qualitative research; the Parse Page, resources for those interested in nursing theory and

Parse's Theory of Human Becoming; and the NURSENET Page, resources for the NURSENET Listserv subscribers.

Contact: Judy Norris, Judy.Norris@ualberta.ca

W Juvenile Diabetes Foundation International (JDF)– The Diabetes Research Foundation

http://www.jdfcure.com/about.htm

JDF's main objective is to support and fund research to find a cure for diabetes and its complications. JDF's site offers diabetes information and news updates, research, and membership information. Celebrity Mary Tyler Moore introduces the home page.

Contact: info@jdfcure.com

W Kent State University School of Nursing

http://www.kent.edu/nursing/nursing.htm

Kent State University School of Nursing was established in 1967. It offers one of the most comprehensive programs of study in nursing in Ohio. It is the largest school of nursing in Ohio and ranks in the 98th percentile in size in the United States. The school enjoys a reputation for excellent academic performance, clinical knowledge, and leadership abilities of its students and graduates. This site is also the home for the *Online Journal of Issues in Nursing.*

Contact: Peggy Doheny, PhD, RN, pdoheny@kent.edu

W Kentucky Coalition of Nurse Practitioners and Nurse Midwives

http://www.achiever.com/freehmpg/kynurses/#kcnpnm

The Kentucky Coalition of Nurse Practitioners and Nurse Midwives is extremely active in its mission to provide services to practitioners and midwives. Each April, the Coalition sponsors a well-attended national educational conference, Toward Excellence in Primary Care and Midwifery. The coalition is also active in raising public awareness of practitioners and midwives, promoting communication among ARNPs, advocating for legislation, and advertising career opportunities. Their home page has pointers to nursing resources, medical news, and online publications.

Contact: Kathy Wheeler, FNPKathy@aol.com

Kirkhof School of Nursing, Grand Valley State University

http://www.gvsu.edu/~nursing/index.html

Information on the School of Nursing, its programs, courses, and faculty. You can take a virtual tour of the school. The faculty listing includes photos, research interests, and courses taught in the past year.

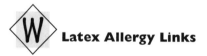 **Knowledge Base: Online Research Methods Textbook**

http://trochim.human.cornell.edu/kb/kbhome.htm

"The Knowledge Base is an online textbook for an introductory course in research methods. I could have written this to read like a regular text, but that would have been boring for me (and probably for you) and there are lots of 'typical' research methods books available now anyway. I thought I would use this new medium to develop a text with a slightly different tone, one that is less formal, more subjective, and perhaps gives the student some insight into how at least one researcher views the area of methodology." Be sure to check out the decision matrix at http://trochim.human.cornell.edu/ojtrial/ojhome.htm to learn more about Type I and Type II errors. Developed by William Trochim at Cornell University.

Contact: William Trochim, wmt1@cornell.edu

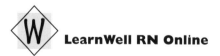 **Latex Allergy Links**

http://pw2.netcom.com/~nam1/latex_allergy.html

A comprehensive site on latex allergy and related links throughout the Internet.

Contact: Nancy, nam1@ix.netcom.com

 LearnWell RN Online

http://www.learnwell.org/~edu/rnonline.shtml

A site with continuing education courses that can be taken online. It is possible to mail in your results to receive CE credit, or just take the courses for personal interest.

Contact: Rudolph Klimes, edu@learnwell.org

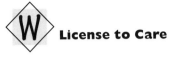 **License to Care**

http://www.nurseid.com/indexa.html

This Website acts as a sounding board for the nursing community. Please share your stories, frustrations, and hopes with them. They are dedicated to promoting the licensed nurse in the age of managed care, downsizing, and deskilling. You can order the RN and LPN lapel pins worn on ER and Chicago Hope at this site.

Contact: donmennig@nurseid.com

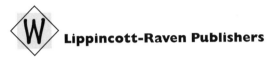 **Lippincott-Raven Publishers**

http://www.lrpub.com/

Lippincott-Raven Publishers is a world leader in information resources for nursing, medical, and allied health professionals and students. For over 200 years, the Lippincott name has become synonymous with nursing education for students, faculty, and practicing nurses. Texts explore modern nursing issues such as health care reform, community-based practice, patient and family teaching, cultural diversity, and others. Lippincott-Raven is a multimedia company. In addition to textbooks, the Lippincott nursing imprint publishes journals, videos, audiocassettes, interactive video discs, and CD-ROMS, offering students new and valuable ways to learn. Lippincott is the publisher of *Computers in Nursing,* the only journal dedicated to nursing informatics.

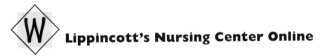 **Lippincott's Nursing Center Online**

http://www.nursingcenter.com or www.agn.org

The former AJN Online has expanded and offers a wide variety of information, including the tables of contents of Lippincott-Raven nursing publications, such as the *American Journal of Nursing, Computers in Nursing, Nursing Research,* and *MCN: American Journal of Maternal Child Nursing,* and books, videos, and multimedia products. A stop here will give the visitor product and subscription information, pointers to electronic discussions, and news. Continuing education is available with instant results. Be sure to check out the nursing treasures section.

Contact: Karen DuBois, karen.dubois@ajn.org

Liszt

http://www.liszt.com

If you are looking for a mailing list, check Liszt. This searchable database includes more than 84,000 entries, with descriptions and subscription information.

 LNCNURSE

LNCNURSE@ontosystems.com

Discussion group for legal nurse consultants.

Type "subscribe" (no quotes) in the subject line of the message.

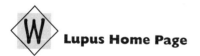 **London Health Sciences Centre**

http://spin.lhsc.on.ca/research/innovati/pathways/

Clinical or critical pathways is a patient management tool that supports continuous quality improvement, efficient resource utilization, and quality patient care. The development of clinical pathways at London Health Sciences Centre was driven by several key goals: to decrease resources and increase health care demands; to maintain high quality, patient-centered care; and to reduce length of stay. A starter kit for implementing clinical pathways has been developed by the center to assist patient care teams and health care organizations embarking on the task of developing clinical pathways.

Contact: wendy.schneidmiller@lhsc.on.ca

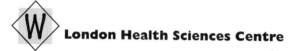 **Lupus Home Page**

http://www.hamline.edu:80/~lupus/

This is a very comprehensive lupus resource, which includes information on lupus mailing lists, searching the lupus Website, and sections on the disease and possible complications. Visitors can also access news updates, abstracts, conference information, and contact information for lupus organizations.

Contact: lupus@piper.hamline.edu

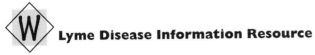 **Lyme Disease Information Resource**

http://www.sky.net/~dporter/lyme1.html

A distributed encyclopedia of information about Lyme disease, covering everything from basic prevention information to research articles. The personal side of the disease is captured in an area called the "Patient Gallery," a small collection of poems and jokes (eg, "Top Ten Things Not to Say to a Lyme Patient") submitted by Lyme disease sufferers.

Contact: Donna Herrell, dporter@solar.sky.net

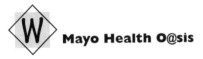 **MacNursing**

http://community.net/~sylvan/MacNursing.html

MacNursing, Sylvan Rogers', RN, contribution to nurses' home pages, features patient databases, care plan generators, hospital unit managers, and nursing resources all for Macintosh computer systems. Visitors can download software and link to other nursing sites.

Contact: Sylvan Rogers, sylvan@community.net

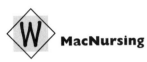 **Mayo Health O@sis**

http://www.mayohealth.org

A multifaceted online health information service sponsored by the Mayo Clinic. There are articles on cancer, diet and nutrition, cardiac disease, women's health, and more. A helpful search feature allows you to easily find resources of interest.

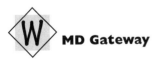 **MD Gateway**

http://www.mdgateway.com/

This site provides daily news and information updates in health care; reviews of medical Internet resources; a learning center; links to publications; and databases of associations, conferences, and manufacturers.

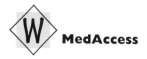

MedAccess

http://www.medaccess.com

A general all-purpose health and medical resource, with many links and lots of helpful resources. Listings of hospitals, patient education materials, news releases, and health quizzes are just a few of the resources available.

Contact: webmaster@medaccess.com

Medical College of Georgia School of Nursing

http://www.mcg.edu/son/index.html

A stop here will deliver information about the school's academic programs, faculty, departments, curriculum, and research efforts. There are also links to other resources within the school. This site includes an informative section on Alzheimer's disease, developed from research conducted by the school of nursing faculty.

Contact: Gregory Bechtel, GBechtel@mail.mcg.edu

Medical Informatics at McGill University

http://mystic.biomed.mcgill.ca/

A site with a wide variety of medical informatics links and information, including an interactive teaching site for breast disease.

Contact: Zs Bencsath-Makkai, zsuzsi@biomed.mcgill.ca

Medical Informatics Laboratory

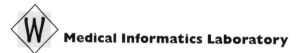

http://ipvaimed9.unipv.it/

Home page of the Medical Informatics Laboratory at the University of Pavia, Italy. Includes descriptions of ongoing research projects in knowledge-based systems and artificial intelligence.

Contact: webmaster@aim.unipv.it

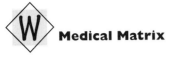 **Medical Matrix**

HTTP://www.medmatrix.org/Index.asp

Ranked, peer-reviewed, annotated, and updated clinical medicine resources. An extremely comprehensive listing can be found at this site. It does require free registration.

Contact: Gary Malet, MD, gmalet@healthtel.com

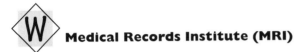 **Medical Records Institute (MRI)**

http://www.medrecinst.com/

MRI works to educate the public about the benefits and hurdles of electronic health records, to support the industry and developers in their efforts, to educate providers about their options in migrating toward electronic health record systems, and to provide information to other parties involved in the process. MRI communicates this message through newsletters, publications, seminars, conferences, symposia, and developers' programs, as well as by participating in applied research and standards work in select areas of interest.

Contact: cust_service@medrecinst.com

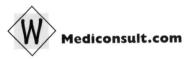 **Mediconsult.com**

http://www.mediconsult.com/

Mediconsult.com is a "virtual medical center" providing quality, patient-oriented medical information and moderated support to patients, families, and health care professionals. Access to the site is free. Information and services are available for more than 50 medical topics.

Contact: Barbara Hansen, ask_barb@mediconsult.com

 MED-JOKES

majordomo@list.pitt.edu

Medical humor and jokes. Can be crude—do not subscribe if you are easily offended.

Subscribe MED-JOKES

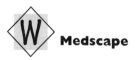 **Medscape**

http://www.medscape.com/

Medscape features regularly updated medical articles and columns. Membership in Medscape is approaching 400,000 reading 300,000 articles a month from a database of almost 10,000 full-text articles in 15 clinical topic areas. There are four varieties of interactive cases in the Exam Room, a small but growing set of tools in the Reference Center, a Continuing Medical Education curriculum, 15 contributing Journals, a growing list of Professional Partners, a bookstore, and MEDLINE integrated with full-text searches. New users are required to fill out a brief registration form (no cost) before they can access full-text articles.

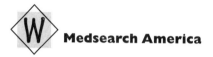 **Medsearch America**

http://www.medsearch.com

Medsearch America is a complete medical recruitment resource offering job seekers a free resumé database, health care job listings, online health care career articles, career resources, and more. Medical or health care job seekers pay nothing for the service.

Contact: webmaster@medsearch.com

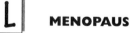 **Men in American Nursing History**

http://www.geocities.com/Athens/Forum/6011/index.html

A slide show that tells the story of men in American nursing history.

Contact: Bruce Wilson, wilson@hiline.net

L   **MENOPAUS**

listserv@psuhmc.hmc.psu.edu

Discussion list on menopause and related women's issues.

Subscribe MENOPAUS Firstname Lastname

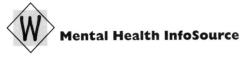
Mental Health InfoSource

http://www.mhsource.com/

An online community for mental health, this site includes patient and professional information, news, continuing education, and consultation.

Contact: Heather Orey, webmaster@mhsource.com

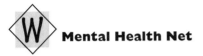
Mental Health Net

http://www.cmhc.com/

Welcome to Mental Health Net, the largest and most comprehensive guide to mental health online, featuring more than 6,000 individual resources. This friendly and fun site covers everything from disorders, such as depression, anxiety, panic attacks, chronic fatigue syndrome, and substance abuse; to professional resources in psychology, psychiatry, and social work; journals; and self-help magazines.

Contact: webmaster@cmhc.com

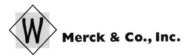
Merck & Co., Inc.

http://www.merck.com/

Merck's Website gives an overview of the pharmaceutical company's major divisions, annual reports, FAQs, research, and product information. One particularly useful feature at this site is the classic *Merck Manual of Diagnosis and Treatment.* The entire manual is online and can be easily searched.

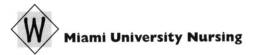
Miami University Nursing

http://www.sas.muohio.edu/nsg/

This home page from the Department of Nursing at Miami University in Ohio has information about its programs, faculty, and courses. In addition, the site features project work by its students, including a very interesting and informative section on dementia.

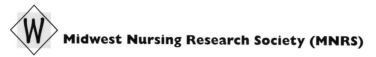

Midwest Nursing Research Society (MNRS)

http://www.mnrs.org/

The Midwest Nursing Research Society is an organization devoted to the development and utilization of nursing research in all health care service and educational settings throughout the 13-state region of the Midwest. The MNRS Website provides information on nursing research, funding sources, publications, program meetings, and information about the MNRS.

Contact: info@mnrs.com

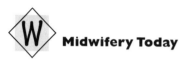

Midwifery Today

http://members.aol.com/midwifery/index.html

Information on publications, educational materials, and conferences sponsored by *Midwifery Today*. Includes information for authors and full text of selected articles.

Contact: midwifery@aol.com

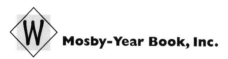

Morbidity and Mortality Weekly Report

http://www.cdc.gov/epo/mmwr/mmwr.html

This report uses the .PDF file format, and to view it you must have Adobe or Acrobat Reader, which can be downloaded. This site gives instructions on how to do this. At this site, the CDC has *MMWR* reports indexed from 1993 to the present for searches on specific topics.

Contact: mmwrq@cdc.gov

Mosby-Year Book, Inc.

http://www.mosby.com/Mosby/index.html

Mosby is a leading publisher of books, journals, and serial publications in the health sciences—medicine, nursing, allied health sciences, dentistry, veterinary medicine—and selected college disciplines—health, physical education and recreation, nutrition, and chemistry. Mosby's Web page contains catalogs, customer support, conference and seminar updates, and online services.

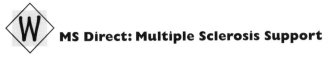 **MS Direct: Multiple Sclerosis Support**

http://www.aquila.com/dean.sporleder/ms_home/

Pointers to multiple sclerosis resources on the Internet, compiled by Dean Sporleder. In his introduction to the page, Sporleder writes, "We can all use different forms of information and hopefully from that info some support. Thanks, and I hope this helps others too."

Contact: Dean Sporleder, msdirect@aquila.com

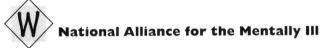 **Multimedia Medical Reference Library**

http://www.mmrl.com/medlibrary/

Jonathan Tward's library of medicine-related Internet sites. The library earns its "multimedia" moniker by pointing users to medical image, movie, sound recording, and software sites.

Contact: Jonathan Tward, jtward@tiac.net

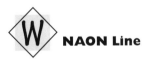 **NAON Line**

http://www.inurse.com/~naon/

Home page of the National Association of Orthopedic Nurses.

Contact: naon@mail.ajj.com

National Alliance for the Mentally Ill

http://www.nami.org

The National Alliance for the Mentally Ill (NAMI) home page offers extensive information about mental illness. The NAMI mission is to "eradicate mental illness and improve the quality of life of those affected by these diseases." To this end, the NAMI site offers information on different disorders, medications, and current research, supplemented by a number of book reviews, and conference and meeting calendars.

Contact: NAMIofc@aol.com

National Alliance of Breast Cancer Organizations

http://www.nabco.org/

"Welcome to the home page of the National Alliance of Breast Cancer Organizations! NABCO is the leading non-profit central resource for information about breast cancer and a network of more than 370 organizations that provide detection, treatment and care to hundreds of thousands of American women. This site will provide you with current information about breast cancer, updates on breast cancer–related events and activities, and links to other Internet sites."

Contact: NABCOinfo@aol.com

National Association for Home Care

http://www.nahc.org/

Home page for the National Association of Home Care, with information on membership, meetings, conferences, news, and legislative and regulatory issues. Includes a listing of state associations.

Contact: webmaster@nahc.org

National Association of Associate Degree Nursing

http://www.podi.com/adnursing/

Home page of N-OADN, the leading advocate for associate degree nursing education practice. The association promotes collaboration in charting the future of health care education and delivery.

Contact: noadn@noadn.org

National Association of Neonatal Nurses

http://www.nann.org/

Home page of the National Association of Neonatal Nurses, the only association in the United States specifically for nurses in this specialty.

Contact: nann84@aol.com

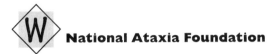

National Association of School Nurses, Inc.

http://www.vrmedia.com/nurses/

Home page of the National Association of School Nurses, Inc., with information on the organization, membership, conferences, and materials available for purchase.

Contact: NASN@mail.vrmedia.com

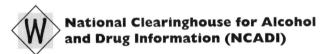

National Ataxia Foundation

http://www.ataxia.org/

The National Ataxia Foundation is a nonprofit organization established in 1957 with the primary mission of encouraging and supporting research into hereditary ataxia, a group of chronic and progressive neurologic disorders affecting coordination. There are more than 45 affiliated chapters and support groups throughout the United States and Canada. This page lists chapter contact information, upcoming events, publications, and support groups.

Contact: NAF@mr.net

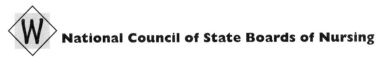

National Clearinghouse for Alcohol and Drug Information (NCADI)

http://www.health.org/

This Website is a service of the Center for Substance Abuse Prevention, Substance Abuse and Mental Health Services Administration, U.S. Public Health Service, and the U.S. Department of Health and Human Services. Visitors will find news, referrals, publications, statistics, forums, databases, a calendar of events, related links, and information about NCADI.

Contact: webmaster@health.org

National Council of State Boards of Nursing

http://www.ncsbn.org/

The NCLEX people. News, information, and links to state boards of nursing.

Contact: webmaster@ncsbn.org

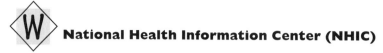

National Health Information Center (NHIC)

http://nhic-nt.health.org/

The NHIC is a health information referral service that puts health professionals and consumers who have health questions in touch with those organizations that are best able to provide answers. NHIC was established in 1979 by the Office of Disease Prevention and Health Promotion (ODPHP), Office of Public Health and Science, Office of the Secretary, U.S. Department of Health and Human Services. The NHIC Health Information Resource Database includes 1,100 organizations and government offices that provide health information on request. Entries include contact information, short abstracts, and information about publications and services the organizations provide.

Contact: NHICinfo@health.org

National Hospice Organization

http://www.nho.org/

Founded in 1978, the National Hospice Organization is the oldest and largest nonprofit public benefit organization devoted exclusively to hospice care. NHO is dedicated to promoting and maintaining quality care for terminally ill persons and their families, and to making hospices an integral part of the U.S. health care system. This site has information about the organization, membership, and locations of hospices throughout the United States.

Contact: Webmaster, DRSNHO@cais.com

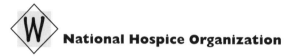

National Institute of Diabetes and Digestive and Kidney Disease (NIDDK)

http://www.niddk.nih.gov/

The National Institute of Diabetes and Digestive and Kidney Disease (NIDDK) is part of the National Institutes of Health (NIH). NIH is the biomedical research arm of the federal government. Based in Bethesda, Maryland, NIH is one of the health agencies of the Public Health Service, which is part of the U.S. Department of Health and Human Services. NIDDK has information on diseases of other types including endocrine, urologic, nutrition and obesity, and hematologic disorders. There are also pointers to information for researchers, news, and other governmental sources of information.

Contact: Kathy Kranzfelder, kranzfeldk@hq.niddk.nih.gov

National Institute of Neurological Disorders and Stroke (NINDS)

http://www.ninds.nih.gov/

NINDS, an agency of the federal government and a component of the National Institutes of Health and the U.S. Public Health Service, is a lead agency for the congressionally designated Decade of the Brain and the leading supporter of biomedical research on disorders of the brain and nervous system. A stop here will render general information on neurologic disorders, a link to available publications, and a database of voluntary health agency contact information.

Contact: Juan M. Munoz, NINDSwebmaster@nih.gov

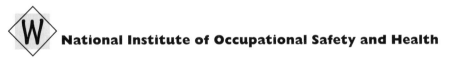

National Institute of Nursing Research (NINR)

http://www.nih.gov/ninr/

NINR's mission is to promote science that strengthens nursing practice and improves health care. NINR supports interdisciplinary research and research training in universities, hospitals, and research centers across the country and conducts intramural investigations at NIH. There is a link to the NINR/Clinical Center Department sponsored Nurse Scientist Training Program, and there is contact information for the NINR's major areas of concentration. The site also has a useful link to schools of nursing throughout the United States, organized by state.

Contact: info@opae.ninr.nih.gov

National Institute of Occupational Safety and Health

http://www.cdc.gov/niosh/homepage.html

This home page has been established to provide information about NIOSH and related activities. The services of NIOSH are available for you to access at the click of the mouse pointer. From these pages you are able to walk inside NIOSH, by subject or category, and find information and services. There are numerous health and safety publications, in both English and Spanish.

Contact: pubstaft@cdc.gov

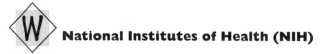

National Institutes of Health (NIH)

http://www.nih.gov/

Any Internet-traveling health professional should plan a stop at the NIH Website. The NIH home page offers news and events; health information; grants and contracts; scientific resources; and links to other institutes and offices, including the National Institute of Nursing Research and the W.G. Magnuson Clinical Center Nursing Department. NIH is a good all-around resource for nurses from all specialties.

Contact: nihinfo@od31tm1.od.nih.gov

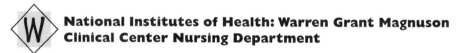

National Institutes of Health: Warren Grant Magnuson Clinical Center Nursing Department

http://www.cc.nih.gov/nursing/lsnn.html

For a complete listing of National Institutes of Health resources, start your journey at http://www.nih.gov/home.html. For a more nursing-specific list of resources, the nursing department page has links to nursing and health-related Websites maintained by universities, the Centers for Disease Control and Prevention, and the National Institute of Nursing Research. There are also links to federal resources, Internet search engines, and other useful resources.

Contact: bbrown@nih.gov

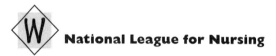

National League for Nursing

http://www.nln.org

This site is a resource center for nursing practice, nursing education, and nursing research. Here you will find features offering you the latest information about NLN membership, Constituent Leagues, accreditation, testing services and tests, and meetings and workshops.

Contact: nlnweb@nln.org

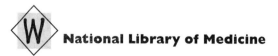

National Library of Medicine

http://www.nlm.nih.gov/

This URL will introduce you to the National Library of Medicine's World Wide Website. Every significant program of the library is represented, from medical history to biotechnology. Visitors here will find news, information about NLM, and its services. Users can access NLM databases and publications and keep up-to-date on research activities, grants, and contracts.

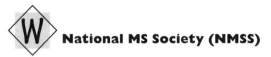

National MS Society (NMSS)

http://www.nmss.org/home.html

NMSS is dedicated to advancing the cure, prevention, and treatment of multiple sclerosis and to improving the lives of those affected by the disease. Visitors to the NMSS site will find information on multiple sclerosis, resources, NMSS, and local chapters, and opportunities to get involved. There is also a link to the National Institute of Health Neurology Institute.

Contact: info@nmss.org

National Network of Libraries of Medicine (NN/LM)

http://www.nnlm.nlm.nih.gov/

Start at the NN/LM for program and resource notes, health-related federal agencies, and other health links. Search NN/LM, accessing resources for medical librarians by U.S. region and research funding resources, and connect to Internet GratefulMed.

National Rehabilitation Information Center (NARIC)

http://www.naric.com/naric

NARIC is a library and information center covering disability and rehabilitation. Funded by the National Institute on Disability and Rehabilitation Research (NIDRR), NARIC collects and disseminates the results of federally funded research projects. The collection, which also includes commercially published books, journal articles, and audiovisuals, grows at a rate of 300 documents a month. NARIC currently has more than 46,000 documents on all aspects of disability rehabilitation.

Contact: Dan Wendling, wendling@macroint.com

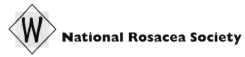 **National Rosacea Society**

http://www.rosacea.org/home.html

Home page for the National Rosacea Society, with information on this condition, educational materials, and other resources.

Contact: rosaceas@aol.com

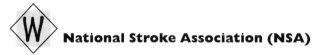 **National Stroke Association (NSA)**

http://www.stroke.org/

National Stroke Association (NSA) is the only national voluntary health care organization focusing 100% of its resources and attention on stroke prevention, treatment, rehabilitation, research, and support for stroke survivors and their families. The largest provider of stroke-related materials in the world, NSA is dedicated to reducing the incidence and impact of stroke by changing the way stroke is viewed and treated. NSA's home page lists educational offerings, facts about and risks associated with stroke, membership information, and volunteer opportunities.

Contact: bleist@stroke.org

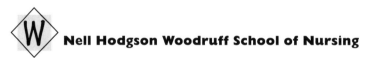 **Nell Hodgson Woodruff School of Nursing**

http://www.emory.edu/WHSC/NURSING/nursing.html

The Nell Hodgson Woodruff School of Nursing is the professional collegiate nursing school of Emory University in Atlanta, Georgia, and is one of seven divisions constituting the Robert W. Woodruff Health Sciences Center. A visitor here will find the school's mission; goals; and information on the academic programs, faculty, and enrollment.

Contact: nurln@nurse.emory.edu

L **NEONATAL-TALK**

neonatal-talk@liststar.bizjet.com

Discussion list for nurses and health professionals in neonatal care.

To subscribe, send a message to the above address with the word "subscribe" (no quotes) in the subject line. Leave the body of the message blank.

NEPHRO-RN

majordomo@majordomo.srv.ualberta.ca

Discussion list for health professionals interested in topics related to nephrology and transplantation.

Subscribe NEPHRO-RN (Note: do not include your name or e-mail address!)

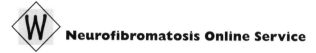 **Neurofibromatosis Online Service**

http://www.nf.org/

Presented by the National Neurofibromatosis Foundation, this page has detailed information on Type 1 and Type 2 of the genetic disorder, neurofibromatosis. Major headings introduce a set of information for patients and one for health care professionals. The patient information covers the basic issues of the symptoms, diagnosis, and genetics of neurofibromatosis. The section for health care professionals covers the more technical issues, such as molecular biology, mode of inheritance, and diagnostic criteria. This page also has information on support groups, online resources, and an overview of the National Neurofibromatosis Foundation.

Contact: Sjouke Zwanenburg, szwanenburg@keep.touch.ch

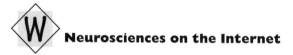 **Neurosciences on the Internet**

http://www.neuroguide.com/

Neurosciences on the Internet contains a searchable index of neuroscience resources available on the World Wide Web and other parts of the Internet. Neurobiology, neurology, neurosurgery, psychiatry, psychology, cognitive science sites, and information on human neurological diseases are covered. Check out the Best Bets page for some excellent links.

Contact: Neil A. Busis, nab@neuroguide.com

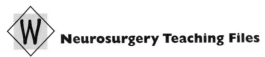 **Neurosurgery Teaching Files**

http://www.neuro.hscsyr.edu/teachfile/teachtop.html

Tutorial on how to take a history, anatomy review, common neurologic emergencies, and more, all presented by the Department of Neurosurgery at Syracuse University.

Contact: Gary Rodziewicz, rodziewg@vax.cs.hscsyr.edu

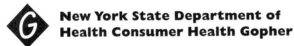 **New York State Department of
Health Consumer Health Gopher**

gopher://gopher.health.state.ny.us/11/.consumer/.factsheets

This Gopher contains fact sheets on various diseases and their causes, symptoms, and treatments.

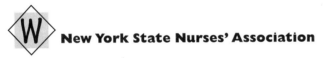 **New York State Nurses' Association**

http://www.nysna.org/

Home page of the New York State Nurses' Association, with membership information, continuing education, economic and general welfare news, governmental affairs, and more.

Contact: info@nysna.org

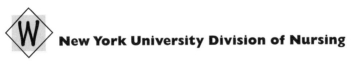 **New York University Division of Nursing**

http://www.nyu.edu/education/nursing/

This Website has information on the academic program, faculty, research programs, and continuing education. It has a nice listing of faculty research with abstracts. There are also nursing links and a pointer to special announcements.

Contact: Barbara Carty, carty@is2.nyu.edu

NIAID (National Institute of Allergy and Infectious Disease) Gopher Server

gopher://odie.niaid.nih.gov/11

The NIAID Gopher Server provides a wide variety of information appealing to both the researcher and the administrator. It has links to the most up-to-date information resources, concentrating on research and reference tools. Of special interest is the AIDS information directory, which contains NIAID press releases, Centers for Disease Control daily AIDS summaries, NIAID protocol recruitment sheets, and many more items of an AIDS or HIV nature.

Contact: Derrick White, gopher@gopher.niaid.nih.gov

NicNet: The Nicotine and Tobacco Network

http://tobacco.arizona.edu

An index ("NicNet Resources") to the smoking resources on the Net, maintained by the Arizona Program for Nicotine and Tobacco Research. Among sites in the index are the University of Pennsylvania's collection of smoking, tobacco, and cancer documents, and a U.S. Department of Health and Human Services pamphlet called "Check Your Smoking I.Q." There is also a set of links to general and health sciences indexes with material on smoking.

Contact: jshober@ccit.arizona.edu

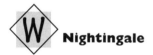

Nightingale

http://nightingale.con.utk.edu/index.htm

This is a WWW site located at the University of Tennessee, Knoxville. Nightingale was one of the first Internet offerings that focused on nursing. Everything you find here will pertain to nursing. Nightingale encourages feedback and contributions to this Website.

Contact: mackbo@utk.edu

NIH-Guide to Grants and Contracts Database

http://www.nih.gov/grants/guide/index.html

The NIH guide is distributed weekly via e-mail to sites that require information about NIH's activities. This site provides a searchable archive of the complete

NIH Guide to grants and contracts. It is also possible to browse each weekly issue of the Guide at this site.

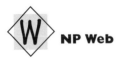 ### NOAH: New York Online Access to Health

http://www.noah.cuny.edu/

New York Online Access to Health (NOAH) is your guide in Spanish and English to the latest health information and resources from volunteer and local governmental agencies, and from other health sites on the Internet. NOAH has information on a wide variety of topics, including aging, AIDS, alternative medicine, cancer, diabetes, healthy living, heart disease and stroke, nutrition, personal health, pregnancy, sexuality, sexually transmitted diseases, and tuberculosis. There is also patient information and a listing of health care organizations in New York state.

Contact: webmaster@noah.cuny.edu

Northern California Nursing Informatics Association (NCNIA)

http://www.dnai.com/~mmoore/ncnia.html

NCNIA is a group of Northern California nurses (and nonnurses) who are interested in issues surrounding the use of computers and software in nursing practice and, more generally, in health care as a whole. NCNIA is a very informal group; it serves primarily to educate its members and provide a forum for discussion of issues that pertain to the practice of nursing informatics specialists.

Contact: mmoore@dnai.com

NP Web

http://www.npweb.org

NP Web is designed to be a tool nurse practitioners may use to improve the use and access of electronic medical resources. As public Internet access improves, and the use of the WWW increases, nurses in advanced practice—whether student, educator, researcher, or seasoned clinician—will be able to use NP Web as a default home page from which to access all resources relevant to practice—virtual one-stop surfing.

Contact: Timothy Cox, RNC, MSN, FNP, tpac@npweb.org

 NP-Clinical

majordomo@nurse.net

Clinical practice issues for nurse practitioners. Nonclinical issues can be discussed on NPINFO.

Subscribe NP-Clinical Your e-mail address

 NPINFO

majordomo@nurse.net

Discussion list for nurse practitioners.

Subscribe NPINFO Your e-mail address

 NP-Students

majordomo@nurse.net

Discussion list among nurse practitioner students, newly graduated nurse practitioners, and nurse practitioner mentors and faculty.

Subscribe NP-Students Your e-mail address

 NRSINGED

listserv@ulkyvm.louisville.edu

Discussion list on nursing education, primarily for educators.

Subscribe NRSINGED Firstname Lastname

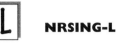 **NRSING-L**

listserv@library.ummed.edu

Discussion list on nursing informatics maintained by Gordon Larrivee.

Subscribe NRSING-L Firstname Lastname

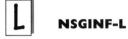 **NSGINF-L**

LISTSERV@LISTS.PSU.EDU

Discussion list for nursing informatics.

Subscribe NSGINF-L Firstname Lastname

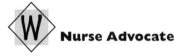 **Nurse Advocate**

http://home.earthlink.net/~carriel/

"Dedicated to the recognition and resolution of workplace violence experienced by nurses; in support of those who have experienced violence; and in memory of those who have died."

Contact: Carrie Lybecker, RN, carriel@earthlink.net

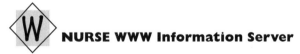 **NURSE WWW Information Server**

http://medweb.bham.ac.uk/nursing/

Includes links to a wide range of nursing resources on the Internet. A new electronic journal, *Nursing Standard Online,* was launched from this site on April 3, 1996. The site is maintained at the Department of Nursing Studies, School of Medicine, University of Birmingham, UK.

Contact: Denis Anthony, cudma@csv.warwick.ac.uk

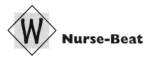

Nurse-Beat

http://badman.drafx.com/Nurse-Beat/

Online cardiac nursing journal, with "Strip of the Month," case studies, and more.

Contact: Debra Kumar, RN, BSN, BA, nurse-beat@drafx.com

NurseLRC

majordomo@douglas.bc.ca

Discussion list for nursing Learning Resource Center faculty and staff to network about psychomotor skill acquisition, care and maintenance of equipment, instructional strategies, computer and audiovisual resources, and funding sources.

Subscribe NurseLRC (Note: do not include your name or e-mail address.)

NURSENET

listserv@listserv.utoronto.ca

A global forum for discussion of nursing issues, maintained by Judy Norris.

Subscribe NURSENET Firstname Lastname

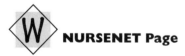

NURSENET Page

http://www.ualberta.ca/~jrnorris/nursenet/nn.html

The NURSENET Page is designed to accompany the Listserv, NURSENET. Includes stats on NURSENET, archives of interesting NURSENET discussions, and educational resources about the Internet.

Contact: Judy Norris, Judy.Norris@ulaberta.ca

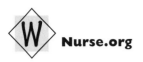 **Nurse.org**

http://www.nurse.org/index2.html

This site is a venture of Nurse Practitioner Support Services of Kent, Washington. It provides information on nursing organizations by state, a listing of state boards of nursing, and employment opportunities.

Contact: Webmaster@nurse.org

 NURSERES

listserv@kentvm.kent.edu

Discussion list on nursing research and related issues.

Subscribe NURSERES Firstname Lastname

 NURSE-ROGERS

mailbase@mailbase.ac.uk

A discussion list for nurses from around the world to enter into scholarly debate and discuss latest developments and significant issues related to Martha Rogers' conceptual system, the Science of Unitary Human Beings.

JOIN nurse-rogers Firstname Lastname

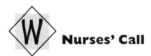 **Nurses' Call**

http://www.nurses-call.org/

This nursing resource has conference announcements, employment opportunities, and a Who's Who in nursing Internet circles. Visitors can also subscribe to nursing Listservs online from this page. You will find contact information for all of the state boards of nursing in the United States, including Guam, Puerto Rico, and the Virgin Islands, as well as Canada, New Zealand, and the United Kingdom.

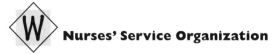

Nurses' Service Organization

http://www.nso.com

Nurses' Service Organization (NSO) is a provider of liability insurance for professional nurses. This site has information on their products. In addition, it includes the current and back issues of the *NSO Risk Advisor*, a newsletter with articles on legal and liability issues.

Contact: NSO_webmaster@aon.com

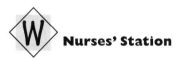

Nurses' Station

http://www.hci.net/~nursecline/

"Welcome to the Nurses' Station. This Website is designed by a nurse for nurses. With health care reform, managed care, and restructuring, or downsizing, taking place in most of the hospitals today, nurses are being placed in even more dangerous and liable positions than previously. This site will, hopefully, give nurses a place to find information on subject matter pertinent to their nursing practice."

Contact: Joseph A. Cline, RN, BSN, nursecline@hci.net

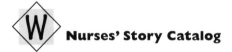

Nurses' Story Catalog

http://web.indstate.edu/nurs/nscat.htm

Nurses' Story Catalog is an Aesopic teaching assistant for nursing teachers, student nurses, nurses, and nurse researchers. Aesop, as you will recall, taught by telling stories that had points and wise sayings associated with them. This teaching method is in contrast to Socrates, who taught by asking questions. Stories transmit information in a situation-specific framework, are easier to remember, pique interest in dry subject matter, operationalize general rules, and illustrate concrete applications of abstract principles. Julia M. Fine of the Indiana State University School of Nursing maintains this page. She welcomes submissions from nurses to add to her database of stories.

Contact: Julia M. Fine, nufine@befac.indstate.edu

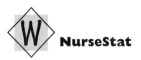 **NurseStat**

http://www.nursestat.com/

"NurseStat is proud to welcome you to the home page of the premiere source for comprehensive nursing information on the Internet for allied health professionals and the general public. Through this web community we encourage everyone to explore our broad range of services and resources and use this knowledge to stretch the bounds of nursing."

Contact: Will Fowlkes, wfowlkes@sios.com

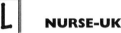 **NURSE-UK**

majordomo@bham.ac.uk

Discussion list for nurses in the United Kingdom.

Subscribe Nurse-UK

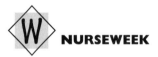 **NURSEWEEK**

http://www-nurseweek.webnexus.com

NURSEWEEK is an online publication devoted to nursing. NURSEWEEK's mission is to support and promote the value of nursing by maintaining a forum for the exchange of information and ideas. The publication reports on local, regional, and national issues from a nursing perspective. It provides health care news, resources, and opportunities to help readers excel in their daily work and reach their career goals.

Contact: chriss@healthweek.com

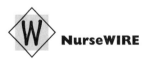 **NurseWIRE**

http://ideanurse.com/nursewire/

NurseWIRE is a service that lists nurse entrepreneurs on the Internet. As the World Wide Web becomes more available and widely used, more nurses in business will find it useful to "hang a shingle" here. Let these enterprising nurses know that you saw them on the Internet!

Contact: Peter Ramme, peter@silicon.com

Nursing and Health Care Resources on the Net

http://www.shef.ac.uk/~nhcon/

A comprehensive list of links for all aspects of nursing. Rod is a nurse in the United Kingdom, so there is a wealth of international information available.

Contact: Rod Ward, Rod.Ward@Sheffield.ac.uk

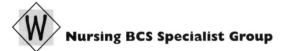 **Nursing and Patient Care Services Duke University Medical Center**

http://nursing-www.mc.duke.edu:80/nursing/nshomepg.htm

The N&PCS site facilitates and shares news, information, and research within the department and DUMC, and provides outreach with the global nursing and health care community.

Contact: N&PCS Web Administrator, goodw010@mc.duke.edu

Nursing BCS Specialist Group

http://www.bcs.org.uk/siggroup/sg39.htm

The Nursing Group of the British Computer Society contributes to national and international debates on information management and technology. The group seeks the views of members through focus groups and links with other bodies within the United Kingdom and with international bodies, such as the International Nursing Informatics Society (INIS) and the European Federation for Medical Informatics (EFMI).

Contact: Carol Cooper, carol.cooper@man.ac.uk

Nursing: Caring for Those in Need

http://www.geocities.com/HotSprings/4709/

Home page of Eric M. Zielinski, RN, BSN. Includes a feature of the month, interactive survey, the nurse's prayer, and more.

Contact: Eric M. Zielinski, RN, BSN, nurse1@geocities.com

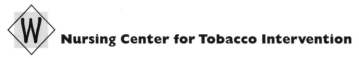
Nursing Center for Tobacco Intervention

http://www.con.ohio-state.edu/tobacco/

This site was created by Mary Ellen Wewers, PhD, RN, and Karen Ahijevych, PhD, RN, of the Ohio State University College of Nursing. They believe that nurses are effective providers of tobacco cessation interventions. Their overall purpose at this site is to increase nurse provider participation in the delivery of tobacco cessation interventions with all tobacco users. Education, information, a forum for interchange, and information on timely topics are all available here.

Contact: ncti@osu.edu

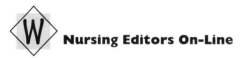
Nursing Editors On-Line

http://members.aol.com/suzannehj/naed.htm

This is an index of nursing journal and book editors. Query them online about your manuscript idea. The editors are listed alphabetically by the title of the journal they edit. You can scroll down, or you can use the "find" feature in your Web browser to locate the editors you want. Each e-mail address has a direct mail link, so all you need is one click on the e-mail address to link with them.

Contact: Suzanne Hall Johnson, suzannehj@aol.com

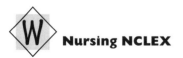
Nursing Mothers' Association of Australia (NMAA)

http://avoca.vicnet.net.au/~nmaa/

The goal of the NMAA is to provide information for both breastfeeding women and for health professionals and others who are involved in supporting and promoting breastfeeding. Visitors here can find out more about this organization and access articles from the Lactation Resource Centre.

Contact: Jenny Gigacz, jgigacz@ozemail.com.au

Nursing NCLEX

http://www.kaplan.com:80/nclex/

This site is sponsored by Kaplan Educational Centers, a company that delivers review courses for the NCLEX licensing examination for nurses. Although there is some commercial emphasis at this site (ie, trying to recruit students for their courses), there are also helpful articles on nursing careers, job opportunities, and graduate education in nursing. If you go to the general home page, there are many links to other educational and testing materials, such as the GMAT, MCAT, GRE, and so forth.

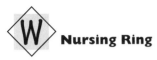 **Nursing Ring**

http://www.geocities.com/Heartland/Plains/2769/nursingring.html

If you have a Website devoted to nursing and want to get the word out to other nurses, consider joining the Nursing Ring. Details on how to do so are available at this site.

Contact: Jeanie, bruce.jeanie@worldnet.att.net

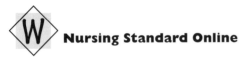 **Nursing Standard Online**

http://www.nursing-standard.co.uk/index.html

Nursing Standard Online gives a selection of articles and abstracts from this week's issue of *Nursing Standard.* Further details on all of their other journals, conferences, and continuing education opportunities are available at the site.

Contact: nso@nursing-standard.co.uk

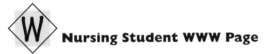 **Nursing Student WWW Page**

http://www.csn.net/~tbracket/htm.htm

Information and resources for nursing students throughout the world.

Contact: Tim Brackett, Tim.Brackett@uchsc.edu

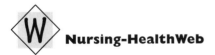 **Nursing-HealthWeb**

http://www.lib.umich.edu/hw/nursing.html

This page is a collaborative effort of the Taubman Medical Library, the School of Nursing at the University of Michigan, and the CIC Health Sciences Internet Working Group. From this page, nurses can connect to career information, clinical nursing resources, interactive forums, academic programs, professional associations, electronic journals, and the HealthWeb.

Contact: nursingpage@umich.edu

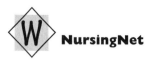 **NursingNet**

http://www.nursingnet.org/

NursingNet was created to help further the knowledge and understanding of nursing for the public and to provide a forum for medical professionals and students to obtain and disseminate information about nursing and medically related subjects. This information includes, but is not limited to, student nursing, specialty nursing, health care issues, and insurance issues. NursingNet offers a chat room, an automated forum, links to other nursing-specific sites, and monthly features.

Contact: nursgnt@nursingnet.org

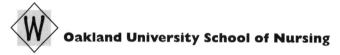 **Oakland University School of Nursing**

http://www.nursing.oakland.edu/

The School of Nursing at Oakland University offers undergraduate and graduate programs designed to prepare nurses to practice in the continuously changing health care system of today and tomorrow. This site includes general information about their programs. In addition, they are developing archives related to Dorothea E. Orem's Self-Care Deficit Theory of Nursing and Imogene King's Open Systems Model. Bibliographies of readings for both theories are available at this site.

Contact: Gary Moore, moore@oakland.edu

 OB-GYN-L

listserv@obgyn.net

Discussion list for obstetrics, gynecology, and related issues. Professionally oriented.

Subscribe OB-GYN-L Firstname Lastname

 Obsessive Compulsive Disorder Resource Center

http://www.ocdresource.com/

The information on this site is offered to inform patients and health care professionals about obsessive-compulsive disorder (OCD)—what it is and what kind of medical treatment and emotional support is available. The site was created with input from OCD patients and medical experts. The site is sponsored by Pharmacia & Upjohn and Solvay Pharmaceuticals.

 ## OCD (Obsessive Compulsive Disorders) Home Page

http://fairlite.com/ocd/

The obsessive-compulsive disorders (OCD) page is a good example of using the Web to create a community. Maintainers Mark and Kelly Luljak (Mark is an OCD sufferer) create an aura of compassion and optimism that is reflected in the postings to the OCD page's popular public bulletin board, the cornerstone of the site. The depth of the information resources available is also impressive; visitors will find personal narratives, medical articles, medication information, and links to other OCD-related sites on the Web.

Contact: fairlite@iglou.com

OCD-L

listserv@vm.marist.edu

Discussion group on obsessive-compulsive disorder.

Subscribe OCD-L Firstname Lastname

Ohio State University College of Nursing

http://www.con.ohio-state.edu:80/

Here a visitor will find general information, as well as nursing, medical, computing, and Internet resources. There are also pointers to the Health Science Colleges and the OSU home page. This site also links to the Nursing Center for Tobacco Intervention, which is affiliated with the college of nursing.

Contact: brownfield.3@osu.edu

OHN-LIST

listserv@oise.utoronto.ca

Discussion list for occupational health nurses and allied professionals.

Subscribe OHN-LIST

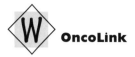 **OncoLink**

http://www.oncolink.upenn.edu

OncoLink is the first multimedia oncology information resource placed on the Internet. OncoLink's mission is consistent with that of the University of Pennsylvania Medical Center and the University of Pennsylvania Cancer Center, which has sanctioned its use and development. OncoLink is accessible worldwide to anyone with Internet access, and there is no charge for its use. OncoLink has been established with the following objectives: (1) dissemination of information relevant to the field of oncology; (2) education of health care personnel; (3) education of patients, families, and other interested parties; and (4) rapid collection of information pertinent to the specialty.

Contact: editors@oncolink.upenn.edu

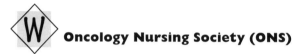 **Oncology Nursing Society (ONS)**

http://www.ons.org

The Oncology Nursing Society has developed the "Netpage" for use by the oncology nurse. Limited information is available at this site for people who are not members of ONS.

Contact: customer.service@ons.org

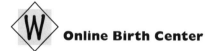 **Online Birth Center**

http://www.efn.org/~djz/birth/birthindex.html

A comprehensive source of information on pregnancy, birth, and breastfeeding. Includes articles, patient information, breastfeeding resources, lists of midwives, a parent's page, information on high-risk pregnancies, and more.

Contact: Donna Dolezal Zelzer, djz@efn.org

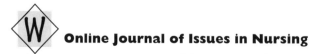 **Online Journal of Issues in Nursing**

http://www.nursingworld.org/ojin/

The purpose of the *Online Journal of Issues in Nursing* is to provide a forum for nurses and other interested parties to exchange opinions and data about topics that affect nursing practice, research, and education. The advantage of having the journal online is that there are no printer delays or space limitations and feedback can be published quickly. Susan L. Jones, PhD, RN, FAAN, is the editor.

Contact: Susan L. Jones, PhD, RN, FAAN, SJonesOJIN@compuserve.com

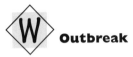

On-Line Journal of Nursing Informatics

http://milkman.cac.psu.edu/~dxm12/OJNI.html

The aim of the *On-Line Journal of Nursing Informatics* (OJNI) is to publish peer-reviewed, original, high-quality scientific papers, review articles, practice-based articles, and databases related to nursing informatics.

Contact: Dee McGonigle PhD, RNC, FACCE, dxm12@psu.edu

Outbreak

http://www.outbreak.org/cgi-unreg/dynaserve.exe/index.html

Outbreak is an online information service addressing emerging diseases. You can search the site as a registered or nonregistered visitor. More information is available to the registered guest, and there is no charge to register.

OVARIAN

listserv@maelstrom.stjohns.edu

A discussion group devoted to ovarian cancer.

Subscribe OVARIAN Firstname Lastname

Pan American Health Organization

http://www.paho.org

This site presents information about the activities, publications, and services of the Pan American Health Organization, an international public health agency based in Washington, DC. The most useful areas are the news releases and the Country Health Profiles, an encyclopedia of the conditions and health concerns of every country in the Americas. A Spanish-language version of this site is also available.

Contact: webmaster@paho.org

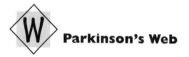 **Parent's Page**

http://www.efn.org/~djz/birth/babylist.html

This page is a resource for parents-to-be, as well as parents of infants and small children. The Parent's Page is a good starting place for links to organizations, multimedia, mailing lists, and health resources that specialize in pregnancy and birth. There is also information about and connections to home-birth and mid-wifery resources as well as adoption, family planning, infertility, and grief and loss.

Contact: Donna Dolezal Zelzer, djz@efn.org

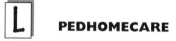 **Parkinson's Web**

http://pdweb.mgh.harvard.edu

There is a vast amount of information about Parkinson's disease and its treat-ment. The problem is where to find the information you are looking for. The purpose of this site is to serve as a resource directory, pointing you to sources of information. This Website is not intended to become a huge repository for all in-formation about Parkinson's. However, with everyone's help, the hope is to guide people to the resources they are seeking.

Contact: pdweb@cisco.com

L **PARSE-L**

listserv@listserv.utoronto.ca

Discussion group related to Parse's Theory of Human Becoming.

Subscribe PARSE-L Firstname Lastname

L **PEDHOMECARE**

listserv@library.ummed.edu

Discussion group for pediatric home care.

Subscribe PEDHOMECARE Firstname Lastname

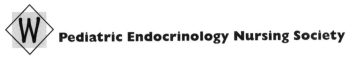

Pediatric Endocrinology Nursing Society

http://ourworld.compuserve.com/homepages/penspage/penspage.htm

Home page for PENS, with newsletter articles, conference information, membership resources, and more.

Contact: penspage@compuserve.com

PEDIATRIC-PAIN

mailserv@ac.dal.ca

Pediatric pain discussion group.

Subscribe PEDIATRIC-PAIN Firstname Lastname

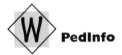

PedInfo

http://www.uab.edu/pedinfo/index.html

This Web server, located at the University of Alabama at Birmingham Division of General Pediatrics and Adolescent Medicine, is dedicated to the dissemination of online information for pediatricians and others interested in child health. There are many links to pediatric resources for parents, nurses, and physicians. There is a Web server search function, research resources, and subscription information for PEDINFO, a pediatric information management Listserv.

Contact: Andy Spooner, spooner@uab.edu

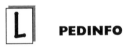

PEDINFO

listproc@u.washington.edu

Discussion group on pediatric medical informatics.

Subscribe PEDINFO Firstname Lastname Degree

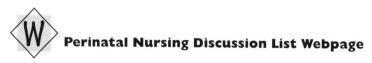

Perinatal Nursing Discussion List Webpage

http://wings.buffalo.edu/academic/department/nursing/mccartny/perintal.htm

Website to accompany the PNATALRN discussion group.

Contact: Patricia McCartney, mccartny@acsu.buffalo.edu

[L] PERIOP

listproc@u.washington.edu

Discussion group for perioperative/OR/theatre nurses worldwide.

Subscribe PERIOP Firstname Lastname

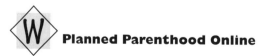

Pets and People: Companion Dogs in Therapy and Service

http://petsandpeople.astraweb.com/index1.htm

Information on service dog training and animal-assisted therapy. Maintained by Pat Gonser, RN.

Contact: pandp@bigfoot.com

PharmInfoNet: Pharmaceutical Information Network

http://pharminfo.com/pin_hp.html

The VirSci Corporation has put together a comprehensive Website for pharmaceutical information. Major headings include news, publications, drug and disease databases, sci.med. pharmacy archives, pharm-mall, job listings, conferences, and related links.

Contact: webmaster@pharminfo.com

Planned Parenthood Online

http://www.plannedparenthood.org

Home page of the Planned Parenthood Association. Includes a newsletter and information on contraception, abortion, parenting, and public affairs. When you enter your zip code, it gives you specialized information on the Planned Parenthood Association in your geographic area.

Contact: communications@ppfa.org

 PNATALRN

listserv@listserv.acsu.buffalo.edu

Discussion group on perinatal nursing practice, education, and research.

Subscribe PNATALRN Firstname Lastname

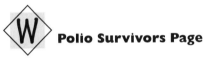 **POLIO**

listserv@maelstron.stjohns.edu

Discussion group for persons affected by polio.

Subscribe POLIO Firstname Lastname

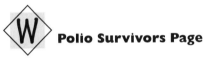 **Polio Survivors Page**

http://www.eskimo.com/~dempt/polio.html

Tom Dempsey has created this page dedicated to persons affected by polio. Visitors will find listings of publications and newsletters on polio, support resources for the disabled, brief biographies of some polio survivors, and links to other polio WWW pages. The site is being maintained collaboratively with the Lincolnshire Post-Polio Network (http://www.zynet.co.uk/ott/polio/lincolnshire/), another resource for post-polio-related information.

Contact: Tom Dempsey, dempt@eskimo.com (Polio Survivors Page) or Chris Slater, linpolioweb@loncps.demon.co.uk (Lincolnshire Post-Polio Network)

 PROSTATE

listserv@maelstron.stjohns.edu

Discussion group for diseases of the prostate.

Subscribe PROSTATE Firstname Lastname

PSYCHIATRIC NURSING

mailbase@mailbase.ac.uk

Discussion group for nurses working in the specialty of psychiatry.

Join PSYCHIATRIC-NURSING Firstname Lastname

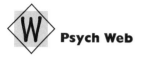 **Psych Web**

http://www.psyche-web.com

This page contains links to noncommercial sites providing information and help about specific disorders related to psychology. In addition to this page, Psych Web maintains lists of brochures and articles related to psychology (many of which are related to self-help issues), commercial psychology–related sites on the Web, other megalists of psychology resources, and scholarly psychology resources on the Web.

Contact: Russ Dewey, rdewey@gasou.edu

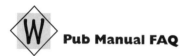 **Pub Manual FAQ**

http://www.apa.org/journals/faq.html

Frequently asked questions for documenting in APA style, prepared by the staff at the American Psychological Association.

 RARE-DIS

listserv@maelstrom.stjohns.edu

Discussion group of rare diseases.

Subscribe RARE-DIS Firstname Lastname

 Registered Nurses Association of British Columbia

http://www.rnabc.bc.ca/

The Registered Nurses Association of British Columbia (RNABC) is the professional organization of all registered nurses and licensed graduate nurses in the province. Everyone wishing to practice as a registered nurse in British Columbia must be a member of the association. Founded in 1912, RNABC's mandate is to serve and protect the public.

Contact: moore@rnabc.bc.ca

 REPRENDO

majordomo@world.std.com

Discussion group for reproductive endocrinology.

Subscribe REPRENDO

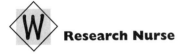 **Research Nurse**

http://www.researchnurse.com

Research Nurse is a journal published 6 times a year to meet the continuing education needs of research practitioners responsible for the conduct of clinical studies. This site hosts the Internet edition of the journal and provides practical information that can be put to use in the day-to-day activities of clinical trials management.

Contact: RN@shore.net

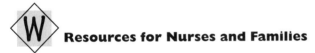 **Resources for Nurses and Families**

http://pegasus.cc.ucf.edu/~wink/home.html

A nice, clean site with resources for families, nurses, and nurse educators. Maintained by Dr. Diane Wink at the University of Central Florida.

Contact: Diane Wink, EdD, RN, wink@pegasus.cc.ucf.edu

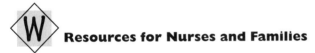 **Revolution: The Journal of Nurse Empowerment**

http://ideanurse.com/advon/

The goal of *Revolution* is to take issue with the "sacred cows" of nursing history—the academic programs that have failed to address the 20th and 21st century concerns—leaving nurses to flounder because curricula have omitted such vital subjects as law, business, ethics, and so forth. The site includes subscription information, general information about the journal, and reprints of past articles.

Contact: Laura Gasparis Vonfrolio, afeduprn@aol.com

 RN Central

http://www.rncentral.com

A place where nurses gather on the Web. Bulletin boards, chat rooms, and resources for students are available at this site.

Contact: Annie Sefic, RN, anniems@earthlink.net

 RN-JOBS

majordomo@npl.com

This list is connected to the Nurses' Call employment pages to provide information concerning professional nursing employment. Users can post employment-wanted information, as well as notices of available positions.

Subscribe RN-JOBS (Note: do not include your name or e-mail address.)

L **RNMGR**

rnmgr-request@cue.com

Discussion group for nurse managers.

Subscribe

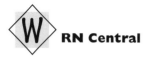 **Robert Wood Johnson Foundation**

http://www.rwjf.org:80/main.html

This sites provides information about the Robert Wood Johnson Foundation—the nation's largest private philanthropy devoted to health care, its programs, and its projects—as well as information about the health care system. Funding information, including listings of current RWJF calls for proposals, open grants, and guidelines for grant applicants, is also available.

Contact: tellus@rwjf.org

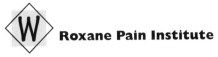 **Roxane Pain Institute**

http://pain.roxane.com/index2.html

This page is sponsored by Roxane Laboratories, makers of Oramorph, a sustained-release form of morphine. The site includes several helpful resources related to pain management including a pain slide show that can be downloaded for teaching purposes. It also includes a complete index to and back issues of the *Palliative Care Letter,* an educational publication with abstracts of articles from scientific publications.

Contact: RPleditor@roxane.com

 RURAL_NURSE

listserv@rhc.org

Discussion group of the Rural Nurse Organization.

Subscribe RURAL_NURSE Firstname Lastname

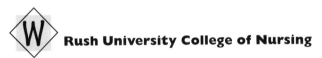 **Rush University College of Nursing**

http://www.rush.edu/RushU/nursing.html

This site provides information on programs within the college, admissions, and organizations. In the faculty section, there is an interesting listing of faculty research projects, with abstracts and references.

Contact: NursingCollege@cnis.rpslmc.edu

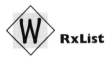 **RxList**

http://www.rxlist.com/

A searchable database of drugs and pharmaceuticals. Search by keyword or imprint ID. The site also includes the top 200 prescriptions by year (amoxicillin was #1 in 1996).

Contact: info@rxlist.com

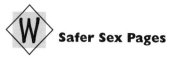

Safer Sex Pages

http://www.safersex.org/

Resource information on safe sex, sexuality, and health. Includes counselor resources.

Contact: ss.admin@safersex.org

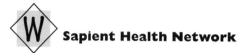

Sapient Health Network

http://www.shn.net

"SHN is an interactive health information service developed for people with chronic and serious illnesses. By providing you with timely information and support, we give you the tools to be your own expert, helping you to make informed decisions about how to fight your disease. Information can make the difference." There are areas on women's health, asthma, breast cancer, heart disease, prostate cancer, and more. Registration is required, but there is no charge.

Contact: support@shn.net

Saskatchewan Registered Nurses' Association

http://www.srna.org/

The Saskatchewan Registered Nurses' Association is the regulatory body for 9,200 registered nurses in the province of Saskatchewan, Canada.

Contact: info@srna.org

SCHLRN-L

listserv@listserv.acsu.buffalo.edu

Discussion group for school nurses.

Subscribe SCHLRN-L Firstname Lastname

School of Nursing at Pennsylvania State University

http://www.hhdev.psu.edu/nurs/nurs.htm

Information on the School of Nursing at Penn State. There is a handy listing of faculty members and their research interests. In addition, a link to the home page of the journal *Qualitative Health Research* can be found at this site. You can also link directly to QHR at http://www.ualberta.ca/~qhr/.

Contact: health@psu.edu

School of Nursing–University of Wisconsin Madison

http://www.son.wisc.edu/~son/index.html

This site includes information on faculty, courses, and programs within the school of nursing. The faculty roster includes pictures, education, research interests, and teaching responsibilities. In the research section, there are narrative descriptions of faculty research and interests.

Contact: Webmaster, rmschust@facstaff.wisc.edu

SCI.MED

The Usenet groups that start with "sci.med" tend to be discussions among health professionals about various health and medical diseases and specialties. Some of the sci.med Usenet groups discuss AIDS, cardiology, ALS, cancer, hepatitis, Lyme disease, orthopedics, and benign prostatic hypertrophy.

Scott's Home Page

http://www.acsu.buffalo.edu/~erdley/

Basically a page of links, but very comprehensive with a little bit of everything. A good place to start a search.

Contact: W. Scott Erdley, RN, MS, erdley@acsu.buffalo.edu

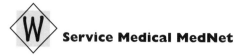

Service Medical MedNet

http://208.140.215.254/sermed/

Service Medical is an independent health care consulting company focused on the development of systems to streamline the product acquisition process and establish internal efficiencies for hospitals. This site has information on the company and links for many other resources.

Contact: gilbert@abelink.com

SERVICE-DOGS

majordomo@acpub.duke.edu

Discussion group for guide, hearing, and assistance dogs.

Subscribe SERVICE-DOGS

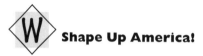

Shape Up America!

http://www.2.shapeup.org/sua/

This Website has been designed to provide the latest information on safe weight management and physical fitness. It includes a cyberkitchen, BMI lab (to calculate body mass index), health and fitness information, and resources designed for professionals.

Contact: suainfo@shapeup.org

Sigma Theta Tau International Nursing Honor Society

http://stti-web.iupui.edu/

Visitors to Sigma's Website can listen to a message from the executive officer, obtain news on members and on the organization, access the *Online Journal of Knowledge Synthesis for Nursing,* access the Virginia Henderson International Nursing Library, and link to chapter Websites.

Contact: Waiping Kam, waiping@stti-sun.iupui.edu

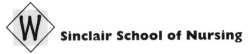
Sinclair School of Nursing

http://www.miaims.missouri.edu/son/docs/sonhome.html

Sinclair's Website has academic program information, a history of the University of Missouri and the school of nursing, and faculty profiles. Visitors can view a quicktime movie, access a calendar of events, and find out about the CNE/Outreach program.

Contact: nursgrid@showme.missouri.edu

SJU Electronic Rehabilitation Resource Center

gopher://sjuvm.stjohns.edu:70/11/disabled

There are two major software archives available through Gopher. The Handicap News BBS Archive and the University of Oakland (Rochester, Michigan) Handicap Archive each contain hundreds of files concerned with all aspects of disabilities and rehabilitation. Both archives can be accessed from the Rehabilitation Resource Center main menu.

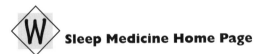
Sleep Medicine Home Page

http://www.cloud9.net/~thorpy/

This home page lists resources regarding all aspects of sleep, including the physiology of sleep, clinical sleep medicine, sleep research, federal and state information, patient information, and business-related groups. Be sure to check out Aristotle's comments on "Sleep and Sleeplessness" from 350 BC.

Contact: thorpy@aecom.yu.edu

SleepNet

http://www.sleepnet.com/

One objective of the SleepNet is to link all known sleep information on the Internet together at one location for easy access. Most answers to questions brought up by this home page can be found on one of the more than 50 links to sleep disorder research centers, support groups, and other organizations devoted to sleep disorders. As they say, "It contains all the answers to the questions you were too tired to ask."

Contact: mesandman@sleepnet.com

| L | **SNURSE-L** |

listserv@listserv.acsu.buffalo.edu

Discussion group for nursing students.

Subscribe SNURSE-L Firstname Lastname

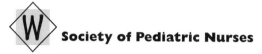 **Society of Pediatric Nurses**

http://www.pednurse.org/

Home page for the society, with membership information, calendar, and more.

Contact: gvargas@aorn.org

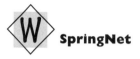 **SpringNet**

http://www.springnet.com/top.htm

This site is brought to you by Springhouse Corporation, publishers of *Nursing98, Nursing Management, Nurse Practitioner,* and the *Nursing98 Drug Handbook.* Visitors to this site can enjoy a wealth of information, including CE offerings, articles, news, a reference library, and career opportunities. There is a wound care center and discussion groups for nurses, nurse managers, nursing students, nurse practitioners, and emergency nurses.

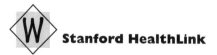 **St. Louis University School of Nursing**

http://www.slu.edu/colleges/NR/

In addition to general information about courses and faculty, this site includes information about the nurse practitioner online distance learning program.

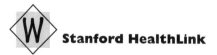 **Stanford HealthLink**

http://healthlink.stanford.edu/

This site includes health and medical news, health tips, and information on medical developments at Stanford University.

Contact: mailbag@healthlink.stanford.edu

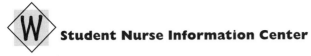 **Student Nurse Information Center**

http://glass.toledolink.com/~ornrsg/

This site is dedicated to providing nursing students with helpful information and links to other resources on the Internet.

Contact: ornrsg@toledolink.com

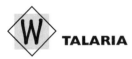 **Sudden Infant Death Syndrome and Other Infant Death (SIDS/OID) Information Web Site**

http://sids-network.org/

This site is the growing collaborative effort of individuals from across the United States and around the world. This sites offers up-to-date information as well as support for those who have been touched by the tragedy of SIDS/OID.

Contact: Chuck Milhalko, sidsnet@sids-network.org.

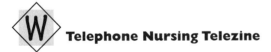 **TALARIA**

http://www.stat.washington.edu/TALARIA/TALARIA.html

A resource for Hypermedia Clinical Practice Guidelines for Cancer Pain. Talaria is a hypermedia World Wide Web implementation of the AHCPR Guidelines on Cancer Pain. Hypertext-linked section headings include: Overview, Assessment of Pain in the Patient with Cancer, Pharmacologic Management, Nonpharmacologic Management: Physical and Psychosocial, Nonpharmacologic Management: Invasive Therapies, Procedure-related Pain in Adults and Children, Pain in Special Populations, and Monitoring the Quality of Pain Management. The site also provides an opioid calculator and links to other cancer sites.

Contact: bradshaw@statsci.com

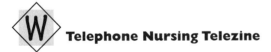 **Telephone Nursing Telezine**

http://www.katsden.com/tnt/index.html

Telephone triage is seen in a variety of settings, including physician practices, health care maintenance organizations, hospitals and clinics, managed care companies, and organized call centers devoted to health information and education. This home page has useful content on telephone triage and dozens of links to other nursing resources.

Contact: Kathi A. Webster, tnt@katsden.com

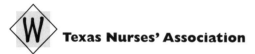

Texas A&M University Corpus Christi School of Nursing

http://www.sci.tamucc.edu/nursing/welcome.html

In addition to the usual information (courses, programs, and faculty), this site has compilations of Internet resources on specific topics, developed by students in the nursing informatics course. A sampling of the topics covered: hay fever, palliative care, stethoscopes, aeromedical evacuation, Alzheimer's caregivers, and sports injuries.

Contact: Whitney Bischoff, DrPH, RN, bischoff@falcon.tamucc.edu

Texas Nurses' Association

http://www.texasnurses.org/

Home page of the Texas Nurses' Association, with membership information, continuing education, legislative news, a members-only chat room, and consumer tips.

Contact: memberinfo@texasnurses.org

Texas Tech University Health Sciences Center School of Nursing

http://www.ttuhsc.edu/pages/nurse/nursing.htm

The Texas Tech School of Nursing was founded in 1981 on the Lubbock campus and expanded to Odessa, Texas, in 1985. The Texas Tech University Health Sciences Center was established in 1971 to serve the citizens of West Texas. This Web page has connections to academic program information, the Nursing Now Newsletter, faculty, advisory committees, and links to nursing Websites.

Contact: Shelley Burson, sonszb@ttuhsc.edu

The Body: A Multimedia AIDS and HIV Information Resource

http://www.thebody.com/

A remarkably comprehensive resource devoted to the myriad facets of the AIDS epidemic, including information on the disease, safe sex, support groups, treatment, mental health, and legal and financial issues. Materials published at the site come from a variety of organizations, both government and private sector nonprofit.

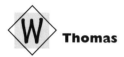 ## Thomas

http://thomas.loc.gov/

Legislative information, brought to you courtesy of the U.S. Congress.

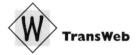 ## TransWeb

http://www.transweb.org/

This site offers insight into organ donation and transplantation. TransWeb features news, a focus on transplant patients, FAQs, links to other transplant resources, and information for health care providers. You can access the International Transplant Nurses Society from this site. (http://www.transweb.org/itns/index.html)

Contact: transweb@umich.edu

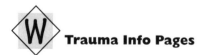 ## Trauma Info Pages

http://gladstone.uoregon.edu/~dvb/trauma.htm

The Trauma Info Pages focus primarily on emotional trauma and traumatic stress, including PTSD (post-traumatic stress disorder), whether following individual traumatic experiences or a large-scale disaster. New information is added once or twice a month. The purpose of this site is to provide information about traumatic stress for clinicians and researchers in the field.

Contact: David Baldwin, dvb@teleport.com

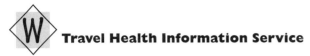

Travel Health Information Service

http://www.travelhealth.com/

"Everything you need for your trip, except the shots!" Lots of information on diseases, vaccinations, food precautions, and other information for people traveling beyond the borders of the United States.

Contact: Stephen Blythe, MD, traveldoc@travelhealth.com

TRNSPLNT

listserv@wuvmd.wustl.edu

A discussion group related to organ transplantation and related issues.

Subscribe TRNSPLNT

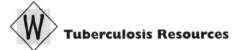

Tuberculosis Resources

http://www.cpmc.columbia.edu/tbcpp/

This page contains information about tuberculosis for the general public and health care providers. Topics for general consumption are the following: what you need to know about tuberculosis, the tuberculin skin test, treatment to prevent tuberculosis, and tuberculosis: getting cured. Health care professionals can view tuberculosis clinical policies and protocols. Content for this page was provided by the Bureau of Tuberculosis Control. This page also has a search function for finding more about tuberculosis within the Web server, and pointers to other tuberculosis resources.

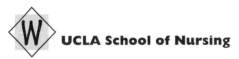

UCLA School of Nursing

http://www.nursing.ucla.edu/

Information about the school and its programs. There is a useful listing of ongoing faculty research.

Contact: James Kimmick, jkimmick@sonnet.ucla.edu

W. U. Massachusetts Medical Center Graduate School of Nursing

http://www.ummed.edu/dept/gsn/index.html

The graduate school of nursing, which offers master's and doctoral degrees, educates clinical nurse specialists and nurse practitioners within three specialties: adult acute or critical care nurse practitioner, adult ambulatory or community care nurse practitioner, and management of nursing practice. This site provides information on all these programs.

Contact: Gordon Larrivee, gordon.larrivee@ummed.edu

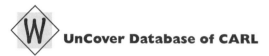 **UnCover Database of CARL**

http://uncweb.carl.org/

UnCover is an online periodical article delivery service and a current awareness alerting service. UnCover indexes nearly 17,000 English language periodicals in its database and is still growing. More than 7 million articles are available through a simple online order system. Five thousand citations are added daily. Articles appear in UnCover at the same time the periodical issue is delivered to your library or local newsstand, which makes UnCover the most up-to-date index anywhere. There is no fee to search the database, but you will be charged for articles you order.

Contact: uncovweb@carl.org

W. United Network for Organ Sharing Transplantation Information Site

http://www.unos.org/

Home page for UNOS, the organization that maintains the Organ Procurement and Transplantation Network. The site includes transplantation statistics, updated weekly.

Contact: webmaster@unos.org

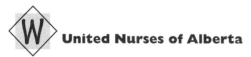 **United Nurses of Alberta**

http://www.ccinet.ab.ca/una/una.html

UNA is a trade union that has represented nurses in Alberta for 20 years and has been instrumental in advancing the profession of nursing. UNA represents 13,500 registered nurses, registered psychiatric nurses, and mental health workers.

Contact: nurses@unab.ab.ca

University of Akron College of Nursing

http://www.uakron.edu/nursing/index.html

This Website has information on the academic program, facilities, international nursing courses, and positions available at the college of nursing. It also includes "The Comfort Line," a section devoted to the concept of comfort in nursing practice and research.

Contact: David Woodruff, dww@uakron.edu

University of Alabama at Birmingham School of Nursing

http://www.uab.edu/son/sonintr2.htm

Home page to introduce the school of nursing, with faculty, course listings, research activities, and more.

Contact: cumminrb@lrc.son.uab.edu.

University of Arizona College of Nursing

http://www.nursing.arizona.edu/

The University of Arizona College of Nursing Website has academic program information, research and scholarship opportunities, and faculty profiles. Visitors can also learn about computer resources and the study abroad program.

Contact: webmaster@www.nursing.arizona.edu

University of Arkansas for Medical Sciences College of Nursing

http://www.uams.edu/nursing/conhome.htm

This site has information on the academic program, continuing education, faculty publications, and a history of the college of nursing. The site has a "virtual tour" of the college of nursing.

Contact: Craig Stotts, rcstotts@con.uams.edu

University of California, San Francisco School of Nursing

http://nurseweb.ucsf.edu/www/ucsfson.htm

Over 500 students enroll each year (from every continent, nation, and region) in the UCSF School of Nursing master's and doctoral programs. The UCSF Nurseweb has information on these programs, the university, news, and employment. A nice, lively site with a variety of information.

Contact: nurosa@itsa.ucsf.edu

University of Central Florida School of Nursing

http://www.cohpa.ucf.edu/nursing/

The School of Nursing offers a bachelor of science in nursing (BSN) program for more than 200 generic and RN-BSN students. The first class of master of science in nursing (MSN) students was admitted in the fall of 1995. This site offers information on programs, admissions, and the campus. It also has a collection of resources to other nursing internet sites and the "Nursing Site of the Month."

Contact: Diane Wink, EdD, RN, wink@pegasus.cc.ucf.edu

University of Colorado School of Nursing

http://www.uchsc.edu/sn/sn/nursing.html

Ranked fifth in the nation in overall excellence, the pace-setting school of nursing enrolls nearly 700 undergraduate and graduate students. Its philosophy—that knowledge of human responses and natural healing processes balances technological advances and biomedical treatments and cures—shapes its programs. This site provides information on the faculty and programs of the school. If you link back to the UCHSC home page, you can connect to the Visible Human Project.

University of Connecticut School of Nursing

http://www.ucc.uconn.edu:80/~WWWNURS/

This site has information on the programs within the school of nursing, the faculty, and the research center. There is an interesting history of the school and a description of the historic Widmer Building, which was recently demolished to make way for a new building.

Contact: Peggy Chinn, plchinn@uconnvm.uconn.edu

University of Illinois at Chicago College of Nursing

http://www.uic.edu/nursing/

Unfortunately, this home page is not terribly well designed. However, if you persevere, you will find a useful listing of faculty and research interests. Information on programs offered by the college is included here as well.

Contact: wchang2@uic.edu

University of Iowa College of Nursing

http://coninfo.nursing.uiowa.edu/index.htm

Home page for College of Nursing at University of Iowa. The research section has excellent links to a variety of projects that are ongoing in the college of nursing, including the Center for Nursing Classification, Family Involvement in Care Study, Gerontological Nursing Interventions Research Center, and more.

Contact: nursing-webmaster@uiowa.edu

University of Kansas School of Nursing

http://www.kumc.edu/instruction/nursing/soninfo.html

The University of Kansas School of Nursing offers a comprehensive curriculum that prepares students for a career in nursing at all levels. The school is known for excellence in critical care, community nursing, and advanced practice nursing, as well as thriving research and diversity programs. This site has links to the virtual classroom—distance learning at KUSON.

Contact: Ivan Bartolome, ibartolo@kumc.edu

W University of Kentucky College of Nursing

http://www.mc.uky.edu/Nursing/

Information on courses, programs, and faculty in the college of nursing. There is a list of faculty research interests and doctoral dissertation titles of their graduates.

Contact: Brenda Ghaelian, brenda@pop.uky.edu

W University of Louisville School of Nursing

http://www.louisville.edu/nursing/

Information on courses, programs, and faculty in the school of nursing. There is a useful list of faculty research interests. On the opening page of the home page is a lovely mosiac representing nursing. Click on it to learn more about its history and meaning.

Contact: Jamie Proctor, jkproc01@homer.louisville.edu

W University of Maine School of Nursing

http://kramer.ume.maine.edu/~nursing/

Information on the school of nursing, faculty, courses, and programs.

Contact: Meg Smith, megsmith@maine.maine.edu

W University of Maryland at Baltimore School of Nursing

http://www.nursing.ab.umd.edu/

The University of Maryland School of Nursing has been a leader in merging technology into nursing learning environments, such as critical care simulation laboratories and interactive laser disc computer simulations. Also leaders in offering interactive video telecourses throughout the state of Maryland, the school is exploring the feasibility of offering state-of-the-art interactive telecourses throughout the world. The school of nursing Web server complements that vision.

Contact: Theodore Stone, tstone@umabnet.ab.umd.edu

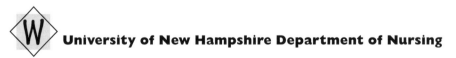

University of Michigan School of Nursing

http://www.umich.edu/~nursing/

Visitors to this home page can read a message from the dean; get information on upcoming events, financial aid, and scholarships; and connect to alumni, faculty, research, and program information. There is also a link to Nursing-Health-Web from this site.

Contact: nursing.web@umich.edu

University of Minnesota School of Nursing

http://www.nursing.umn.edu/

The University of Minnesota School of Nursing was established in 1909 as the first university-based school of nursing in the world. It is part of the university's Academic Health Center, which is dedicated to the improvement of health through the discovery and dissemination of new knowledge. This Website has information on degree programs, the faculty, administrators, and current research.

Contact: hanso041@maroon.tc.umn.edu

University of New Hampshire Department of Nursing

http://unhinfo.unh.edu/nursing/index.html

Home page for the UNH Department of Nursing.

W   University of North Carolina at Chapel Hill School of Nursing

http://www.unc.edu/depts/nursing/

This site includes information on the school of nursing and its programs. In addition, there is a nice description of the Center for Research in Chronic Illness and the research being conducted by nurses in the center.

Contact: nursing@unc.edu

W   University of North Carolina at Greensboro School of Nursing

http://www.uncg.edu/nur/sonhome.htm

The University of North Carolina at Greensboro School of Nursing World Wide Web page is designed to provide information about UNCG School of Nursing programs. The site also includes useful guides to nursing resources on the Internet.

Contact: Ann Martin, martina@florence.uncg.edu

W   University of Pennsylvania School of Nursing

http://www.upenn.edu/nursing/

The University of Pennsylvania is composed of 4 undergraduate and 12 graduate and professional schools that are philosophically and functionally unified on a self-contained, 260-acre campus. This site offers information on the school, its programs, faculty, and research.

Contact: John Kahler, jkahler@pobox.upenn.edu

W   University of Phoenix

http://www.uophx.edu/

University of Phoenix offers graduate and undergraduate degree programs to working professionals around the world. With 51 campuses and learning centers located throughout the United States and the Commonwealth of Puerto Rico, including the Online Degree Program and Center for Distance Education, University of Phoenix is one of the nation's largest private accredited institutions for business and management. This site provides information on its nursing programs, as well as many others.

W University of Pittsburgh School of Nursing

http://www.pitt.edu/~nursing/

Information on the educational programs within the school of nursing are contained at this site. The listing of faculty research interests with photos and inspirational quotes is nicely done.

Contact: nursing+@pitt.edu

W University of Rochester School of Nursing

http://www.urmc.rochester.edu/SON/index.html

A visitor here can get an overview of the school of nursing and its academic programs. Be sure to check out the "Research Fables From the Sisters Grinn," which can be found within the Nursing Research CyberCourse.

Contact: webmaster@miner.rochester.edu

W University of South Carolina College of Nursing

http://www.sc.edu/nursing/

The college of nursing Web page has pointers to administrative and clinical nursing, family and child nursing, faculty, and staff.

Contact: meason@gwm.sc.edu

W University of Southern Maine College of Nursing

http://www.usm.maine.edu/~son/

Information on the college of nursing, the faculty, courses, and programs. The page opens with a beautiful picture of Portland Head Light.

Contact: SON@USM.Maine.edu

University of Tennessee at Chattanooga School of Nursing

http://www.utc.edu/~utcnurse/index.htm

Information on the programs and courses are available at this site. There is a handy listing of faculty with its expertise, research interests, and teaching areas. In addition, projects by students in the MSN program are highlighted.

Contact: Pam Taylor, RN, PhD, Pam-Taylor@utc.edu

University of Texas at Austin School of Nursing

http://www.utexas.edu/nursing

This site has detailed information on the programs, courses, and faculty at the school of nursing. It also includes a listing of all dissertation titles completed by students in the school from 1971 to the present.

Contact: nursing@uts.cc.utexas.edu

University of Texas Health Science Center at San Antonio

http://www.uthscsa.edu/nursing/son_main.htm

"Welcome to our School of Nursing, the largest nursing program in the University of Texas System. The commitment of our faculty is to educate students to function on the cutting edge of technology and patient care, and we have developed innovative courses in all our programs of study. Our current enrollment is 892 students; 546 undergraduate, 200 master's and 46 doctoral candidates. I hope you enjoy your visit with us."

Contact: Elaine Graveley, DBA, RN, graveley@uthscsa.edu

University of Texas–Houston School of Nursing

http://son1.nur.uth.tmc.edu/

This site includes information on the school of nursing, its programs, faculty, students, and research. The link to the Center on Aging has some useful information.

Contact: www@son1.nur.uth.tmc.edu

W University of Texas M. D. Anderson Cancer Center (UTMDACC)

http://www.mdanderson.org/

This site contains information about resources for cancer available from the UTMDACC Cancer Information Service, the Texas Cancer Data Center, and CancerNet.

Contact: www@www.mdanderson.org

W University of Texas School of Nursing at Galveston

http://www.son.utmb.edu/

This site has information on the school of nursing, its faculty, and programs. There are some interesting historical pictures of the university and Galveston. This site also contains the Academic Journal Directory, a very helpful resource for nurse authors (and aspiring nurse authors!).

Contact: Andrew W. Hall, ahall@sonpo.utmb.edu

W University of Utah College of Nursing

http://www.nurs.utah.edu/

The nursing program at the University of Utah became a college of nursing in 1948, awarding the baccalaureate degree to both generic and registered nurse students. The baccalaureate and graduate programs are fully accredited by the National League for Nursing. The college is the only PhD nursing program in the state of Utah to prepare nursing faculty. This Website details these programs.

Contact: webmaster@nightingale.nurs.utah.edu

W University of Virginia School of Nursing

http://www.med.virginia.edu/nursing/NurseHome.html

This home page contains a message from the dean, academic program information, descriptions of the research and academic centers, faculty profiles, and links to other nursing Internet resources.

Contact: cb5e@virginia.edu

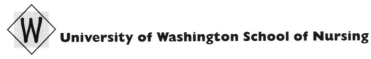

University of Washington School of Nursing

http://www.son.washington.edu/

The University of Washington offers four degree programs: the BSN, MN, MS, and PhD. This page has academic program information and connects to the school's three departments: Biobehavioral Nursing and Health Systems, Family and Child Nursing, Psychosocial and Community Health. If you connect to the main home page of the university (http://www.washington.edu), you will see a live picture of the campus—on sunny days, you can see Mt. Rainier in the background!

Contact: webster@son.washington.edu

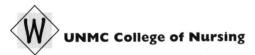

University of Wisconsin–Milwaukee School of Nursing

http://www.uwm.edu/Dept/Nursing/

The mission of the School of Nursing of the University of Wisconsin–Milwaukee reflects the primary mission of a university: to generate knowledge through research and practice, and to disseminate knowledge through graduate and undergraduate programs, continuing education, and public service. This Website describes nursing academic programs, faculty, research, continuing education, and employment opportunities.

Contact: Beth Rodgers, brodg@csd.uwm.edu

UNMC College of Nursing

http://www.unmc.edu/c_nursing/

At the University of Nebraska Medical Center College of Nursing site you will find information on courses, programs, and online continuing education. In addition, the site has a searchable database to identify research interests of all 800 faculty (not just nursing) at the university. It is possible to search by name or keyword.

Contact: cedmunds@netserv.unmc.edu

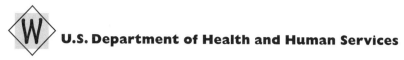

U.S. Department of Health and Human Services

http://www.dhhs.gov/

Information about the mission of the U.S. Department of Health and Human Services (HHS), plus HHS publications and press releases and links to other government health and medicine resources on the Net.

Contact: webmaster@os.dhhs.gov

USUHS–Uniformed Services University of the Health Sciences

http://www.usuhs.mil/

The Uniformed Services University of the Health Sciences is the nation's federal health sciences university and is committed to excellence in military medicine and public health during peace and war. USUHS provides the nation with health professionals dedicated to career service in the Department of Defense and the United States Public Health Service and with scientists who serve the common good. It serves the uniformed services and the nation as an outstanding academic health sciences center with a worldwide perspective for education, research, service, and consultation; it is unique in relating these activities to military medicine, disaster medicine, and military medical readiness. This site has information on the programs within USUHS, including the graduate school of nursing.

Contact: Alex D. Khuc, webmaster@usuhs.mil

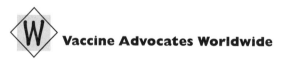

Vaccine Advocates Worldwide

http://www.vactup.org/index.html

Recognizing the urgent need for an effective and affordable HIV vaccine, a group of community members formed VACTUP (Vaccine Advocates Committed to Universal Prevention). The mission is to advocate for accelerated development efforts toward a safe, effective, and affordable HIV vaccine, accessible globally to at-risk populations. This site has information on HIV vaccine development.

Contact: input@vactup.org

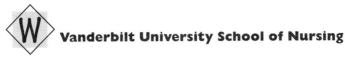 **Vanderbilt University School of Nursing**

http://www.mc.vanderbilt.edu/nursing/

With a history dating back to 1909, Vanderbilt University School of Nursing has an established reputation for excellence in nursing education. This Website has information on academics, admission procedures, research, and the Nashville community.

Contact: Larry Lancaster, larry.lancaster@mcmail.vanderbilt.edu

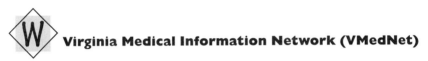 **Virginia Medical Information Network (VMedNet)**

http://vmednet.gen.va.us/

The Virginia Medical Information Network (VMedNet) is an electronic network of Virginia health care providers and information linked via the Internet. Established by the Health Sciences Center at the University of Virginia, VMedNet is meant to serve as a central clearinghouse of clinical and educational resources.

Contact:VMedNet@virginia.edu

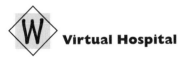 **Virtual Health and Nursing Place**

http://www.algonet.se/~pelundb/

Home page of Peter Lundberg, Swedish nurse, with a little bit of everything. Interesting resources on nursing in Scandinavia.

Contact: Peter Lundberg, pelundb@algonet.se

Virtual Hospital

http://vh.radiology.uiowa.edu/

The Virtual Hospital (VH) is a project of the Electric Differential Multimedia Laboratory, Department of Radiology, University of Iowa College of Medicine. It is a continuously updated digital health sciences library stored on computers and available over high-speed networks 24 hours a day. The VH provides invaluable patient care support and distance learning to practicing physicians and other health care professionals.

Contact: librarian@vh.org

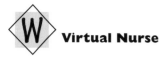 **Virtual Nurse**

http://virtualnurse.com/

A little bit of everything can be found at this site: chat rooms, message boards, funny nursing stories, and more.

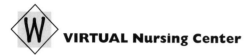 **VIRTUAL Nursing Center**

http://www-sci.lib.uci.edu/HSG/Nursing.html

Martindale's Health Science Guide links to nursing resources categorized as medical dictionaries and glossaries, metabolic pathways and genetic maps, interactive anatomy browsers, online nursing journals, nurses' courses, tutorials and lectures, interactive patient browsers, and general nursing information.

Contact: Jim Martindale, jmartindale@ymsa.oac.uci.edu

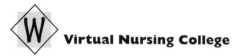 **Virtual Nursing College**

http://www.langara.bc.ca/vnc/

The VNC is a virtual learning and teaching environment that uses concept-resource mapping, multimedia, and full access to Internet and virtual reality. This page offers a comprehensive list of links to nursing research resources, cardiovascular information, images and pathology sites, publications, medical sites, and holistic sites.

Contact: Jack Yensen, jyensen@mail.bc.rogers.wave.ca

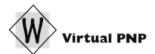 **Virtual PNP**

http://home.earthlink.net/~emgoodman/virtualpnp.htm

A Website for pediatric nurse practitioners and their child and adolescent patients. The site includes case studies, clinical insights, professional links, employment opportunities, and continuing education.

Contact: Eric Goodman, MSN, emgoodman@earthlink.net

Walkers in Darkness

majordomo@world.std.com

Walkers in Darkness is a support list for depression, bipolar disorder, and related mental illnesses and their treatment, coping mechanisms, and recovery techniques. Walkers members comprise a wide variety of backgrounds, levels of functioning, and stages of recovery ranging from newly diagnosed to those who have learned to cope with their illness.

Subscribe walkers (Note: do not include your name or e-mail address.)

Wayne State University College of Nursing

http://www.comm.wayne.edu/nursing/nursing.html

Information on the college of nursing, its programs, courses, and faculty. There is an interesting and detailed description of the Center for Health Research.

Contact: NURINFO@cms.cc.wayne.edu

Web Extension to American Psychological Association Style

http://www.nyct.net/~beads/weapas/

For those of you writing term papers or manuscripts for publication, here is the source that tells you how to document your online references in proper APA style.

Contact: webmaster@beadsland.com

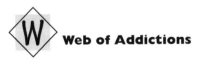 **Web of Addictions**

http://www.well.com/user/woa/

The Web of Addictions is dedicated to providing accurate information about alcohol and other drug addictions. It provides a resource for teachers, students, and others who needed factual information about abused drugs.

Contact: Andrew L. Homer, ahomer@mail.coin.missouri.edu

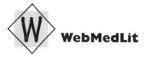 **WebMedLit**

http://www.webmedlit.com/

WebMedLit is a medical headlines service. WebMedLit scans the Web each night for updates to medical journals. All links point back to the original articles or abstracts at the publishers' Websites. In general, the sources followed must provide at least some abstracts to the full-text articles; sites providing only tables of contents are not tracked by WebMedLit. The sources tracked by WebMedLit are primarily concerned with clinical topics or human epidemiology. The site is sponsored by Silver Platter Information, Inc., and the Physicians Home Page.

Contact: feedback@webmedlit.com

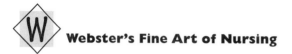 **Webster's Fine Art of Nursing**

http://www.katsden.com/nursing/index.html

A great nursing site created by Kathi Webster, RN. The site is dedicated to her great-great-grandfather, Aaron Webster, who was a nurse stationed near Washington, DC, during the Civil War.

Contact: Kathi Webster, webster@katsden.com

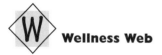 **Wellness Web**

http://wellweb.com/

A resource for health care consumers, with health education information on topics ranging from smoking to heart disease to women's health. For a quick guide to the material available at the site, choose the alphabetical Master Index from the main menu.

Contact: feedback@wellweb.com

WellTech

http://www.welltech.com

The WellTech site is designed to provide online resources for health promotion and wellness professionals. WellTech gathers, develops, and manages health promotion resources from around the world. WellTech's goal is to link health educators, wellness directors, publishers, and health program developers with the information critical to their work.

Contact: info@welltech.com

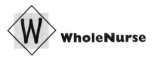 **West Virginia University School of Nursing**

http://www.hsc.wvu.edu/son/

Home page for school of nursing at WVU. Information on "Nursing Workforce Network" is contained at this site.

Contact: Deborah Lewis, dlewis@wvnvm.wvnet.edu

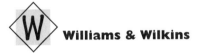 **WholeNurse**

http://www.wholenurse.com/index.html

WholeNurse's vision is to help make sense out of the shifting, intensely growing information base of the Internet for nurses, patients, and medical personnel of all kinds. Read some of the articles, get FAQs on some common diseases, find out about alternative and complementary health care, participate in the WholeNurse Message Board, and see what's happening in the holistic community.

Contact: rlphelps@accesscom.net

Williams & Wilkins

http://www.wwilkins.com/

Williams & Wilkins is a leading international health science publisher with its headquarters at Camden Yards in Baltimore, Maryland. Topics of particular interest from the electronic media catalog include nursing management and administration; critical care nursing; medical, surgical, and home health nursing; mental health nursing; pediatric nursing; and nursing of general interest. Visitors may also want to stop at webROUNDS, an interactive, online journal for medical students; and the Science of Review home page, featuring information on all of the health science admission and licensing exams covered by its Science of Review product line, from the MCAT through the USMLE Step 2.

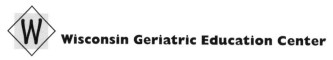

Wisconsin Geriatric Education Center

http://www.marquette.edu/wgec/

The ultimate goal of the Wisconsin Geriatric Education Center (WGEC) is to enhance the quality of life and promote wellness for the elderly in Wisconsin through the stimulation, coordination, implementation, and dissemination of geriatric education for health care faculty and providers. This site provides a variety of information toward accomplishing that goal.

Contact: wgecnet@vms.csd.mu.edu

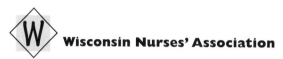

Wisconsin Nurses' Association

http://www.execpc.com/~wna/

Home page of the Wisconsin Nurses' Association, with membership information; STAT bulletins; a nurse practitioner forum; and a listing of Wisconsin politicians, including e-mail addresses.

Contact: imagine@mail.execpc.com

WITSENDO

listserv@caligari.dartmouth.edu

Discussion group on endometriosis.

Subscribe WITSENDO Firstname Lastname

WOMENS-HEALTH

womens-health@obgyn.net

Discussion group on women's health.

Subscribe WOMENS-HEALTH Firstname Lastname

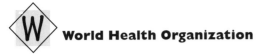 **World Health Organization**

http://www.who.ch

Home page of the World Health Organization, located in Geneva, Switzerland. There is a wealth of information available at this site. A good search engine helps you to quickly access the materials you need.

Contact: webmaster@who.ch

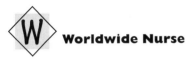 **Worldwide Nurse**

http://www.wwnurse.com/

Developed and maintained by Brian Short, RN, this home page has pointers to other nursing resources, disease links, search forms, and medical software reviews.

Contact: Brian Short bshort@wwnurse.com

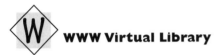 **WWW Virtual Library**

http://vlib.stanford.edu/Overview.html

A distributed subject catalog. There are a number of health and nursing related entries that contain useful links.

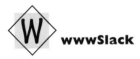 **wwwSlack**

http://www.slackinc.com/wwwslack.htm

Much of the material in wwwSLACK is closely related to its traditionally produced publications. There are descriptions and excerpts from books, abstracts and full articles from its journals, membership services, and public information offerings from client associations.

Contact: webmaster@slackinc.com